KW-054-900

Contents

Illustrations

THE NATURAL WAY

Premenstrual Syndrome

Jane Sullivan

Series medical consultants
Dr Peter Albright MD (USA)
& Dr David Peters MD (UK)

Approved by the
AMERICAN HOLISTIC MEDICAL ASSOCIATION
& BRITISH HOLISTIC MEDICAL ASSOCIATION

ELEMENT
Shaftesbury, Dorset ● Rockport, Massachusetts
Melbourne, Victoria

© Element Books Limited 1996
Text © Jane Sullivan 1996

First published in the UK in 1996 by
Element Books Limited
Shaftesbury, Dorset SP7 8BP

Published in the USA in 1996 by
Element Books, Inc.
PO Box 830, Rockport, MA 01966

Published in Australia in 1996 by
Element Books
and distributed by
Penguin Books Australia Limited
487 Maroondah Highway, Ringwood, Victoria 3134

Reissued 1998

Cover design by Slatter-Anderson
Designed and typeset by Linda Reed and Joss Nizan
Printed and bound in Great Britain

British Library Cataloguing in Publication

Library of Congress Cataloging in Publication Data
Sullivan, Jane.
The natural way with premenstrual syndrome/Jane Sullivan.
p. cm. – (Natural way series)
Includes bibliographical references and index.
ISBN 1–85230–805-X (pbk: alk. paper)
1. Premenstrual syndrome–Popular works 2. Premenstrual syndrome-
-Alternative treatment. I. Title. II. Series.
RG165.S85 1996
618.1'72–dc20   95–44032
CIP

ISBN 1 85230 805 X
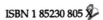

Acknowledgements

Thanks go to the many doctors, natural therapists and nutritionists who helped in the research for this book, and to the women who were so willing to talk about their experiences and who gave a real insight into the world of the PMS sufferer.

Introduction

Premenstrual syndrome, PMS for short, affects millions of women around the world. It's no exaggeration to say that almost every woman will experience some symptoms associated with PMS at least once in her life. For many these are merely a mild irritation – perhaps a headache or feeling more tired – a signal that a period is on its way. But for others the symptoms are more severe. Depression, cravings for sweets, breast pain, aggression are all more serious problems that can play havoc with a woman's life.

For years PMS has been a bit of a Cinderella condition. Doctors labelled women with PMS as 'neurotic' and told them their problems were 'all in the mind'. Countless women have been told to 'pull yourself together' by doctors frustrated at the lack of available treatments for this condition.

Progress in understanding the true causes of PMS has brought a shift in attitude to it – and better treatments. Women with the condition are far less likely to be written off as neurotic cases as doctors now realize that it is a real medical condition. But, as doctors would be the first to admit, conventional medicine does not have all the answers for sufferers. There is no wonder drug for this condition.

One thing that has become abundantly clear is that mind and body cannot be separated when it comes to dealing with PMS. Simply treating the symptoms of PMS is not enough. Understanding and dealing with the mind and emotions is the other side of the story.

This is where many of the natural therapies score points over conventional medical approaches. Their 'holistic' approach of treating the whole person rather than just the disease pays dividends when it comes to PMS. Certainly many women are finding that the gentle approach is more effective than many of the treatments offered by conventional medicine.

This book has been written as a guide to understanding more about the natural therapies. Its aim is to help you to help yourself get better.

CHAPTER 1

What is premenstrual syndrome?

How it happens and who it affects

Premenstrual syndrome – PMS for short – was first recorded in 1931. But despite more than 60 years of research, doctors still have little idea of the causes of a condition that affects millions of women around the world.

Theories have come and gone as often as therapies to treat it.

In the early days, when extreme PMS was considered to be a mental disorder, women were treated with drugs to control depression (*antidepressants*), electric shock or electroconvulsive therapy, and even surgery to cut out a part of the brain (*lobotomy*). Even today some women who have tried every available treatment without success may be offered a *hysterectomy*, an operation to remove the womb and the ovaries, in an attempt to relieve the condition – though this is an absolutely last ditch approach.

Thankfully, no woman need resort to such drastic solutions. If you think you suffer from PMS, there are simple, effective measures that can relieve the condition, even though the cause of it is largely unknown.

Why PMS is described as a 'syndrome'

Premenstrual syndrome (PMS) is now the accepted term for the condition. Previously the term *premenstrual tension*, or PMT, was used but this is inaccurate as tension is not the only symptom that women experience. A syndrome more accurately describes the condition because it means a collection of symptoms. Strictly speaking, the term covers only symptoms that occur in the two weeks before menstruation.

The symptoms of PMS

There are so many symptoms associated with PMS (*see* Figure 1) that diagnosing the condition is not always easy. Some medical textbooks list up to 150 symptoms that have been associated with the condition and many of the symptoms of PMS are also found in other illnesses.

Headache, insomnia, feeling 'low', irritability, and sugar cravings are not only felt by women with PMS. Men, children and women without PMS may all experience these symptoms.

The key definition of PMS, now accepted by most doctors, is that symptoms occur only in the two weeks before a period and that there are absolutely no symptoms for at least seven days after a period has started.

Symptoms tend to fall into two categories: physical and psychological. Given the huge number and range of symptoms associated with PMS, it is not surprising that it is sometimes confused with other conditions. Indeed some conditions, such as depression, may be masked because a woman also has PMS or mistakes her symptoms for PMS.

For this reason it is essential to write down any symptoms that occur throughout the month by keeping some form of diary (*see* box page 7 'Doing your own PMS chart'). No good practitioner would diagnose PMS until a monthly pattern to the symptoms has been established.

Doctors are also reluctant to treat PMS unless the symptoms are severe enough to significantly alter a woman's lifestyle. Many women who experience irritability, or fatigue, or who gain weight before a period will not be diagnosed as having PMS because these symptoms are regarded as normal.

However, that does not mean you have to stand by and do nothing. There is plenty you can do to ease these problems – *see* Chapters 4 and 5 on self-help and beating stress.

Physical symptoms	Psychological symptoms
Breast tenderness	Depression or feeling low
Swelling or bloated feeling	Fatigue, listlessness
Puffiness	Tension/aggression
Weight gain	Irritability
Headache	Clumsiness
Appetite changes	Difficulty in concentrating
Craving for sugar	Decreased or increased
Acne	interest in sex
Constipation or diarrhoea	Mood swings
Stiff muscles or joints	Needing more or less
Abdominal pain or cramps	sleep
Backache	Insomnia
Tiredness	
Worsening of conditions like epilepsy, migraine, asthma	

Fig. 1 The most common PMS symptoms (in approximate order of how frequently they occur)

The positive side of PMS

Yes, there is a positive side. A study of 102 women attending well woman clinics in Toronto, Canada, found that 70 per cent reported at least one good thing when they were premenstrual. This included:

- increased interest in sex (37 per cent)
- tendency to clean or tidy up (32 per cent)
- increased enjoyment of sex (31 per cent)
- a tendency to 'get more things done' (29 per cent)
- more attractive breasts (20 per cent)
- more energy (18 per cent)
- more creative ideas at work (11 per cent)
- performing better at work (8 per cent)
- increased confidence (6 per cent)

Although the positive sides of PMS may not wholly compensate for the negative aspects, it can be helpful to know that PMS is not all bad. The other positive aspect is that, once diagnosed, PMS can be treated effectively.

Who gets PMS?

Anyone from a teenager to a granny may get PMS but it seems to be more common in women in their 30s and 40s – at least that is the age range that most commonly come forward for treatment.

But this does not mean that women not in their 30s can't or don't get PMS. Women in the 45 to 50 age group may experience a worsening of their PMS symptoms or even experience PMS for the first time as they approach the menopause. Whatever the cause, any changes in symptoms needs to be investigated properly as the symptoms of PMS in this age group may be confused with the menopause but the treatments are quite different.

The different types of PMS

Estimates of the number of women with PMS vary widely. Studies around the world have produced figures ranging from 40 to 95 per cent.

But what is clear is that PMS is not the same for everybody. Symptoms range from mild to severe, says Dr Diana Saunders from the University of Oxford in England. She puts women into three categories:

- *Mild PMS* affects 75–90 per cent of women at some time in their life. For these women PMS is not a debilitating condition. They can carry on with their normal routine, at work or at home, without major problems. They may simply feel more tired than usual, or a bit 'down in the mouth' or irritable.
- *Serious PMS* affects around 10 per cent of women. They find the monthly round of PMS symptoms too much to cope with and need help.
- *Severe PMS* affects up to 3 per cent of women. In these cases PMS symptoms are so severe and distressing that they wreak havoc.

Pigeonholing PMS

Some PMS researchers group women according to their type of symptoms. The UK-based Women's Nutritional Advisory Service uses the following system:

- *Type A* is for anxiety symptoms – nervous tension, irritability and mood swings.
- *Type H* is for hydration symptoms – bloating and water retention.
- *Type D* is for depression – uncontrolled crying, feeling down in the mouth or sad, feeling confused, even suicidal.
- *Type C* is for cravings – wanting sugary foods, feeling weak and dizzy if you don't eat them.

As many women can fall into two or even three categories this classification is not widely used.

Risk factors for PMS

Studies of women with PMS show that there are some situations which are associated with a high risk of developing PMS. The most common triggers are hormone upsets:

- childbirth – although PMS may not appear until after the birth of a second or subsequent child
- postnatal depression
- recent gynaecological operations
- miscarriage or abortion
- gynaecological disorders such as endometriosis or ovarian cysts.

In addition there appear to be general lifestyle factors which are linked to PMS. Three important ones are:

- poor diet
- lack of exercise
- stressful events such as illness or relationship problems.

Diagnosis

There is no simple test for PMS. None of the modern medical tests such as blood tests, hair analysis, sweat tests and so on can positively diagnose PMS. Doctors presented with a case of suspected PMS will first try to exclude other diseases that may be the cause of symptoms before labelling the woman as a sufferer.

Can I diagnose myself?

Self-diagnosis of PMS is notoriously unreliable. It is not true that you have PMS simply because you have periods. An accurate diagnosis is only possible if a diary of symptoms has been kept for at least two, preferably three, menstrual cycles and has shown that those symptoms *only* occur before a period and never in the seven days afterwards.

Dr Maureen Dalton, consultant gynaecologist at Sunderland Hospital in the UK and daughter of PMS pioneer Dr Katharina Dalton, says that only 50 per cent of the women who complain of PMS actually have it.

Women tend to remember the time that they lost their temper if their period started the day afterwards whereas at other times of the month they have nothing to help them remember, she says.

Accurate diagnosis is important to avoid incorrect and ineffective therapy. If you have a thyroid disorder, for example, which may cause symptoms similar to PMS such as fatigue and irritability, then you will gain little from therapies designed to relieve PMS.

Doing your own PMS chart

A simple, but effective, chart for recording PMS symptoms is one based on Figure 2. Record your two or three worst symptoms using a simple code for each symptom. For example breast tenderness could be denoted by the letter 'B' and headache by the letter 'H'. You could distinguish between severe and mild symptoms by using a capital letter for severe and a small letter for mild. You must record the days of menstruation.

Give a chart to your husband or partner to fill in as well. At the end of the month see if they match up.

Although you may have more than two or three symptoms it is easier to keep the chart if you simply record your worst symptoms or those which you would like to get rid of first. After a couple of months you will see a pattern beginning to emerge like one of those in Figure 3.

While you are completing the chart it is important to try and keep an open mind and not to try and evaluate your chart before the two or three months are up. Simply record your symptoms, if any, at the end of each day and then forget about the chart until the next day.

Length of cycle	1	2	3	4	5	6	7	8	9	10	11	12	13	14	15	16	17	18	19	20	21	22	23	24	25	26	27	28	29	30	31
Jan																															
Feb																															
Mar																															
April																															
May																															
June																															
July																															
Aug																															
Sept																															
Oct																															
Nov																															
Dec																															

Mark an 'M' for days of your period. Mark the days of your three worst symptoms with an appropriate abbreviation.
eg H = Headache, D = Depression, I = Irritability, B = Breast discomfort, W = Water retention

Fig. 2 PMS symptom chart

(a)

	1	2	3	4	5	6	7	8	9	10	11	12	13	14	15	16	17	18	19	20	21	22	23	24	25	26	27	28	29	30	31
March							M	M	M	M	M	M	M	M	M	M														H	H
April	I,D	I,D	I,D	I,D	I,D	I,D	I,D	M	M	M	M																				

(b)

	1	2	3	4	5	6	7	8	9	10	11	12	13	14	15	16	17	18	19	20	21	22	23	24	25	26	27	28	29	30	31
March			T	T	T	T		M	M	M	M	M	M	M,T	M,D	D	D	D	D						I	I	T,I	T,I			
April			T,D	T,D				M	M	M	M			T,D	T,D	T	T	T													

H = Headache; T = Tiredness; I = Irritability; D = Depression

Fig. 3 a) Symptom chart of woman with typical PMS
b) Symptom chart of woman with no PMS pattern

Why is PMS important?

Research by the British PMS researcher Dr Katharina Dalton has linked PMS with crime, child abuse, car accidents, suicides, school truancy and exam failure. This research is controversial. Some researchers have questioned the thinking that once a month some women become a hazard to themselves and society just because a period is due.

PMS is seldom regarded as a life-threatening condition. But if the symptoms are so severe that a woman is violent towards her children or her partner then the condition must be taken seriously.

There is no doubt that in a few cases PMS can be a disabling and frightening condition. There have been, thankfully rare, cases of women who have committed murder while they were suffering from PMS and this has been used in court as their defence.

Once you have established that your symptoms occur in the premenstrual phase of your cycle and you feel they are bad enough to need some treatment then you have several options open to you.

First, it is wise to find out a little more about the normal menstrual cycle and the hormones involved (Chapter 2).

Then when you know more about your menstrual cycle you can try self-help measures to get to grips with the problem (Chapter 4). Only if those fail will you need to seek help from a medical or natural practitioner (Chapters 6–9).

All about the menstrual cycle

How it works and the hormones that control it

Women today have many more periods than their great-great grandmothers. A girl starting her periods today at around 13 years old can expect to have 400 periods before she reaches the menopause. In Victorian times, according to Dr Alan Riley, a British expert in sexual medicine, women had as few as 40 periods in their life-time. The main reasons for the increase are:

- Girls in the Western world mature earlier than they have ever done before so they start their periods earlier.
- Women today have fewer babies than in the past when a baby every 12 to 18 months was not uncommon.
- Women don't breast-feed as much as their grandmothers did. (Breast-feeding is a natural suppressor of the normal menstrual cycle. Today women breast-feed for only a few months compared with two years or more in times past.)
- Women live longer than they used to. More women are surviving to the menopause then ever before.

It is only since women started having more and more regular cycles that problems such as PMS have become recognized. In the past PMS may not have been so common, or recognized, because women had so few periods. To understand PMS properly it is helpful to understand something of the normal menstrual cycle.

The normal menstrual cycle

Counting the days between the start of each period is the best way to start so that you can find out more about your normal cycle length.

We are taught from girlhood that a normal menstrual cycle is 28 days long – that is 28 days from the start of one menstrual period to the start of another. But 28 days is only an average. In fact only one woman in eight conforms to this standard cycle.

Cycles can vary from 24 to 35 days and it is perfectly normal for a woman to have a 24-day cycle one month and a 35-day cycle the next.

The menstrual cycle is incredibly sensitive to change. Some women find that a holiday can delay their period, or the stress of starting a new job may bring the period on earlier than expected.

Not much is known about how various stresses work to change the length of the menstrual cycle. If your period is late or early then don't worry – it's normal.

No matter how long your cycle, there is one thing that remains constant. Ovulation, the release of a fertile egg from the ovary, always occurs 14 days before the start of your next period.

What controls the menstrual cycle

The menstrual cycle is under the control of four hormones:

- oestrogen
- progesterone
- follicle-stimulating hormone (FSH)
- luteinizing hormone (LH)

Oestrogen and progesterone are responsible for triggering ovulation and building up the lining of the womb in preparation for a pregnancy.

FSH and LH are two hormones called *gonadotrophins*. They are produced by the *pituitary gland* in the brain and control the production of oestrogen and progesterone.

The pituitary gland is controlled by a gland in the brain called the *hypothalamus*. This produces the gonadotrophin-releasing hormone (GnRH) which stimulates the production of FSH and LH from the pituitary.

The phases of the menstrual cycle

The monthly cycle is usually divided into three phases:

- menstruation
- follicular (or proliferative) phase
- luteal (or secretory) phase

Menstruation (days 1–6)
A normal period lasts from one to eight days although the average is five. During menstruation levels of oestrogen and progesterone are at their lowest. This triggers the unfertilized egg and the lining of the womb to be shed, resulting in bleeding.

Follicular phase (days 7–14)
FSH and small amounts of LH are produced by the pituitary gland. This triggers the ovaries to develop several small fluid-filled compartments (called *primordial follicles*) which contain eggs. The follicles produce increasing amounts of oestrogen as they mature.

Oestrogen levels peak just before ovulation and this triggers a surge of LH from the pituitary. The most mature egg at the time of the 'LH surge' is released from the ovary. Ovulation usually occurs within 36 hours of the LH surge.

Once a ripe egg has been released the other follicles degenerate. In the meantime the womb has also been active: its lining thickens and becomes spongy in preparation for pregnancy.

Luteal phase (days 15-28)

The follicle that contained the egg is now called the *corpus luteum*. LH triggers the corpus luteum to produce progesterone which encourages the growth of the extra blood vessels in the womb needed for a pregnancy.

The corpus luteum remains for around 14 days after ovulation when it shrivels up and dies. Progesterone levels fall from around day 22 of the cycle.

Oestrogen levels also fall during this time and, as these hormones fall, the lining of the womb degenerates, so completing the cycle. PMS occurs during the luteal phase of the cycle, after ovulation.

Figure 4 shows the changes in hormone levels during the menstrual cycle.

Hormones and the rest of the body

Oestrogen and progesterone are not only involved in the menstrual cycle. Almost every bodily system is affected in some way or another by one of these hormones.

Oestrogen

There is hardly a part of the body that is not affected by oestrogen. Doctors studying the menopause have discovered that oestrogen is involved in:

- keeping cholesterol levels lower to help protect against heart disease
- keeping bones strong
- keeping skin and hair strong and healthy
- breast development
- controlling our mood and emotions – oestrogen is known to have 50 actions in the brain. It helps with memory function, it is known to be a natural tranquillizer and antidepressant and is often described as the 'happy hormone'. Sexual drive is also linked with oestrogen.

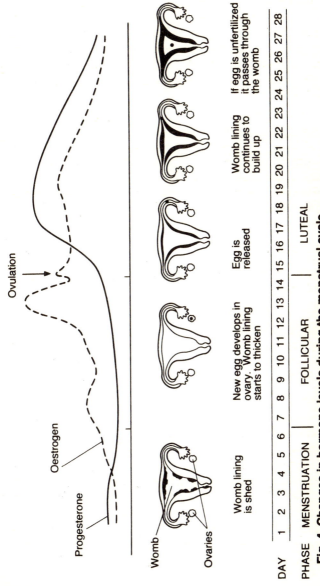

Fig. 4 Changes in hormone levels during the menstrual cycle.

Progesterone

Progesterone also has a far wider impact than simply regulating menstruation. It is involved in:

- sleep mechanisms – healthy volunteers injected with progesterone fall asleep
- controlling blood sugar levels – lack of progesterone leads to cravings for sweet foods which is the body's way of saying its blood sugar has fallen too low
- controlling mood and emotions – in some studies synthetic progesterone has brought on depression within a few hours of being given to healthy people

Although doctors do not know everything about the way hormones work there is very strong evidence that hormones are at the root of PMS. We'll look more at likely causes and triggers of PMS in Chapter 3.

Causes and risk factors in PMS

How and why PMS develops

PMS is controversial because its cause is still shrouded in mystery. For years the idea that PMS is just a sign of a 'neurotic woman' has hampered funding for research. It's only in the last 10 or 15 years that PMS has been taken seriously and that quality research into its cause has begun. This research has proved once and for all that chemical and hormonal factors strongly influence PMS. It is definitely not *'all* in the mind'.

Although it's known that there are biological influences in PMS, quite what they are continues to divide the experts. At the moment research centres on three areas:

- a hormone imbalance
- nutritional deficiencies
- brain chemical disorders

In fact it may turn out that PMS is a combination of all three. At the moment it's a bit of a chicken and egg argument. Which came first – the hormone imbalance or the brain chemical disorder or the nutritional deficiencies? Only further research will provide the answers.

The hormone imbalance theory

It seemed obvious when PMS was first recorded in the medical textbooks that it must have a hormonal cause. Since PMS only occurs during the luteal phase of the menstrual cycle (in the two weeks before a period), research has focused on the hormones at that time of the month.

At this time of the cycle, levels of oestrogen drop markedly, while levels of progesterone are usually fairly high. There are two camps in the hormone debate. One side says that PMS is caused by a lack of oestrogen. The other says that PMS is caused by lack of progesterone.

The oestrogen theory

Support for an oestrogen deficiency has come from studies of women who have had their normal menstrual cycle stopped. Doctors do this either by giving women a drug that blocks the action of GnRH (the hormone that controls the regulation of the menstrual cycle) or surgery to remove the womb and ovaries.

When the menstrual cycle is stopped women do not get PMS. If women are then given oestrogen-replacement therapy they still do not develop symptoms. If, however, they are given progesterone, or its artificial form *progestogen*, they develop PMS-like symptoms.

Doctors who believe that PMS is caused by a lack of oestrogen tend to treat women with oestrogen therapy (*see* Chapter 6).

The progesterone theory

On the other side of the hormone argument are doctors who believe that PMS is caused by a progesterone defect. Dr Katharina Dalton, who runs a clinic treating women with PMS and postnatal depression in Harley Street, London, is a leading proponent of this theory.

She believes that PMS is caused by a lack of progesterone or a defect in the way the body can use the progesterone present. She strongly favours progesterone therapy for severe PMS cases.

According to Dr Dalton the progesterone defect stems from:

- poor eating habits
- stressful lifestyles

Large gaps between meals, she claims, lead to a drop in normal blood sugar levels. Normally that is no problem as the body has a natural mechanism for keeping blood sugar levels steady. It calls on its reserves of glucose stored in the liver and the body cells. To retrieve this glucose the body releases a hormone called *adrenalin* (also known, particularly in the USA, as *epinephrine*).

Problems arise because a byproduct of adrenalin – *noradrenalin* (or *norepinephrine*) – blocks the space on the cell surface that would usually be used by progesterone. It's rather like trying to fit a key into a lock which already has a key in the other side. You won't be able to open the door.

Instead of fitting into its rightful place on the cell surface the progesterone wanders around the body trying to find a cell that will have it. This may explain why women with PMS have normal levels of progesterone in their blood. Their hormone levels are normal but they can't use that hormone.

Another situation in which a lot of adrenalin is released is during times of stress. Not surprisingly, studies of PMS have shown that women report worse symptoms when they are under a lot of stress. (For more about stress *see* Chapter 5.)

To overcome the excess of adrenalin Dr Dalton advocates regular snacks of starchy foods, like wholemeal bread, to avoid low blood sugar. (This will be discussed further in Chapter 4.) If a change of eating habits does not work then Dr Dalton recommends progesterone therapy as it is likely that the body's cells cannot use normal levels of progesterone effectively.

Nutritional deficiencies

There is plenty of research to support a link between poor eating habits and PMS. The main problems are thought to be caused by shortages of:

● vitamins, particularly B-group vitamins
● minerals such as magnesium and zinc
● essential fatty acids

Vitamin and mineral deficiencies

One of the oldest theories to explain PMS is that a deficiency of vitamin B6 is to blame. Vitamin B6 is involved in the production of chemicals in the brain called *neurotransmitters* that are known to be responsible for making us happy.

Low levels of these 'happy chemicals' have been shown to lead to depression. They also trigger an increase in two hormones: *prolactin* and *aldosterone.*

High levels of prolactin cause premenstrual breast pain and tenderness.

Aldosterone triggers the kidneys to reduce the amount of urine they excrete. This means more water is kept in the body leading to bloated abdomen, weight gain and puffiness.

Vitamin B6 supplements have for many years been a mainstay of PMS therapy (*see* Chapter 6) but it is now thought that a combination of vitamins and minerals is more effective in treating PMS because no vitamin or mineral works in isolation in the body. In the case of PMS the effects of vitamin B6 are thought to be enhanced if vitamins B1 and B2 and the minerals calcium, magnesium and zinc are given at the same time.

Lack of essential fatty acids

Essential fatty acids (EFAS) are not fats, like butter, nor acids like those you might have used in school chemistry lessons. They are more like vitamins (in fact they were called vitamin F when they were first discovered). EFAs are vital for good health and, because our bodies cannot make them, we have to obtain them from our food.

EFAs belong to a group of *polyunsaturated fatty acids* (PUFAs for short). PUFAs have several roles in the body including:

- forming part of the membrane that surrounds every cell in the body
- production of a special group of chemicals called *prostaglandins*
- providing energy
- maintaining body temperature
- insulating the nerves

In the case of PMS it's thought that the effect on prostaglandin production is the root of the problem.

There are several types of prostaglandin (scientists believe there are many more that have not yet been discovered). They are involved in a range of processes from blood clotting, lowering blood pressure, causing the womb to contract, and protecting against stomach ulcers.

In the brain a shortage of prostaglandins is thought to lead to low levels of the body's natural tranquillizers, the endorphins – hence the symptoms of anxiety reported by some women with PMS.

The most important source of EFAs in the diet are meats, dairy products, oily fish, seafoods such as shrimps and prawns, and green leafy vegetables.

The main problem for premenstrual women is that Western diets, which are rich in saturated fats and low on vitamins and minerals, block the conversion of the main form of EFA – *linoleic acid* – into a form that the body can use called *gamma-linolenic acid*. Smoking and excess alcohol also block the chemical pathway.

The story is further complicated by the fact that there are two forms of linoleic acid. One of them – the *cis* form – is more easily used by the body than the other – the *trans* form.

The natural state of most PUFAs is in the *cis* form. But during heating or the process of 'hydrogenation' (as, for example, in the manufacture of 'low fat' spreads) the molecule may become changed into the *trans* form.

For the body, trying to use the *trans* form is rather like trying to put a left shoe on your right foot. It looks similar but the 'fit' is wrong.

In effect the *trans* forms are useless as the body cannot convert them and they prevent the body from using *cis* forms as they block the spaces in the cells where the chemical conversions take place. It's rather like the battle for space between adrenalin and progesterone.

Since some processed foods such as soft margarines and vegetable cooking oils (particularly those that contain hydrogenated oils) may contain up to 50 per cent *trans*-fatty acids there is real concern that EFA deficiency is widespread.

Brain chemical disorder

One of the most exciting advances in the last five years has been the discovery of a link between the female hormones and chemicals in the brain called *neurotransmitters* that are responsible for controlling our mood and emotions.

What are neurotransmitters?
Neurotransmitters are so called because they transmit messages from one nerve cell to another. There are several types:

- *Dopamine* is found in the parts of the brain that control movement.

- *Serotonin* is the main neurotransmitter in the parts of the brain that are involved in conscious processes such as thought, emotions, mood and memory.
- *Acetylcholine* is found in muscles where it causes them to contract.
- *Noradrenalin* (which is also a hormone) controls heart beat and blood flow.
- There is also a group of neurotransmitters called *neuropeptides*. These include chemicals such as the endorphins that are involved in controlling pain.

The neurotransmitters most relevant to PMS are serotonin, the brain's so-called 'happy chemical', and endorphins, the body's natural anti-anxiety chemicals.

Serotonin
Support for the role of serotonin in PMS is growing all the time. In early 1995 researchers from the UK Medical Research Council's brain metabolism unit in Edinburgh, Scotland, found that oestrogen stimulates the production of receptors in the brain that respond to serotonin.

The work was carried out on rats who had had their ovaries removed so that they could not produce oestrogen. Half the rats were given a dose of oestrogen and 24 hours later the rats' brains were examined. Brains from the oestrogen-treated rats took up more serotonin – and therefore had more serotonin receptors – than the brains from rats which had not been dosed with oestrogen.

The researchers also discovered that oestrogen increases the activity of a gene that is involved in the production of the serotonin receptor in the brain.

The Edinburgh researchers are currently studying women to see if what happens in rats also happens in humans. This time they are using 'high-tech' brain scans to detect serotonin to see if the density of receptors changes during the menstrual cycle in line with the rises and falls in oestrogen. If oestrogen is found to affect serotonin receptors then it may explain why antidepressant drugs which increase serotonin levels have been shown to treat the anxiety symptoms of PMS successfully.

In fact there is already evidence that serotonin levels are lower in women with PMS. Blood tests have shown lower levels of serotonin in women with PMS than in those without the condition.

American research into the links between the food we eat and our mood further supports the serotonin theory. It has been shown that foods that are high in sugars and starches lead to an increase in a chemical called *tryptophan*, which is converted into serotonin by the body.

It's thought that the monthly craving for sugary foods which some women experience may be the body's way of saying it needs more serotonin. In practice, however, much of the food we eat also contains small amounts of fat which would cancel out the serotonin-boost of the sugar. So, in fact, a binge on sugary snacks is not an effective way of cheering yourself up.

Endorphins
In the 1970s it was discovered that the body had its own natural painkillers which were similar in structure to *morphine* – a drug used to relieve severe pain in cancer patients. These natural painkillers were called 'endogenous morphines', or endorphins for short.

Since their discovery it has been found that endorphins also:

● help control the body's response to stress
● regulate contractions of the intestine
● lift our mood
● regulate the release of hormones from the pituitary gland

In the mid-1980s it was found that women with PMS have low levels of beta-endorphins in the luteal phase of the menstrual cycle. This led to the suggestion that PMS could be a kind of opiate withdrawal syndrome.

According to this concept, women are dependent on their own endorphins and at times of the menstrual cycle, when endorphin levels are low, they experience irritability and depression – a form of 'cold turkey'.

Oestrogen is known to increase levels of beta-endorphins so this may be one reason why women feel all right before ovulation when oestrogen levels are high and experience PMS afterwards when oestrogen is on the decline.

There is also some evidence that endorphin levels are affected by prostaglandins. So if there is a shortage of the necessary prostaglandins there may in turn be a shortage of endorphins.

So which theory is correct?

The answer is that all of them may be correct. One of the emerging themes from PMS research is that the hormones, nutrition and brain chemistry are closely linked. PMS probably has no single cause but may occur when several things go wrong at the same time. A poor diet may lead to low levels of brain chemicals which plummet even lower at times of the month when oestrogen is low.

Or there may be different types of PMS, each with a different cause.

For this reason it is best to keep an open mind towards treatment. Doctors, and women, often become frustrated because there are so many different treatments for PMS. What works for one woman may not work for another. And until the causes of PMS have been completely unravelled PMS therapy will remain a mishmash of different approaches.

The key is to find out what you can do to help yourself and where to go if you cannot cope on your own.

CHAPTER 4

How to help yourself

Tips for prevention and treatment

Recognizing that you have PMS is half the battle in getting to grips with the problem. If you have filled in a symptom chart for at least two months and you feel that your symptoms are due to PMS then there are several things you can do to help yourself before asking your doctor or a natural therapist for help.

The first thing is to take a hard, honest, look at your lifestyle. Do you eat a truly healthy diet? Do you take enough exercise? Do you get enough sleep? For most of us the answer to these questions is 'no', 'no' and 'no'.

Modern living demands a lot of our bodies. We rush out of the house without breakfast to catch a train or sit in a traffic jam to get to work. We spend all morning on the go with endless cups of coffee or tea to keep us going. Lunch might be a rushed snack before more hours sitting behind a desk.

Then it's back home for an evening spent putting children to bed, helping with homework, cooking the evening meal, catching up on the chores or slumping in front of the television before a restless night spent counting sheep or worrying about all the things you haven't done.

If that is the type of life you lead then it will not be long before the cracks start to appear. Whether it's PMS or some other condition, before long your body will rebel and start telling you it has had enough. And if this is the case, it will take more than a pill to put it right.

You will have to change your lifestyle. But in the long term you will reap the benefits in terms of better health, fitness and relief from PMS.

There are three steps you can take on the path back to full health:

- eat a healthy diet
- take more exercise
- reduce your stress (this is so important that it deserves a chapter to itself – *see* Chapter 5)

Most of us know, deep down, that good health depends on a healthy diet and plenty of exercise. But the message bears repeating *because it really does work*. Thousands of PMS sufferers are reaping the benefits of a change of lifestyle. Not only is their general health better but they have cast off the shackles of the monthly PMS misery.

If you want to help yourself, these are safe, non-medical, actions that you can take to benefit your general health and your PMS.

Diet

If you are confused about what is a healthy diet then you are not alone. We are swamped with information about food and often this week's newspaper headline directly contradicts last week's. It's no wonder that we give up and stick to the junk.

However, there is no doubt that the typical Western diet is not regarded as health promoting. Our diets have been transformed in the last 50 years. Today we eat a vast array of foods and snacks that were unheard of when our parents and grandparents were children.

Unfortunately many of these foods are high in fats and sugars and low in important nutrients such as vitamins and minerals. They also tend to have additives such as artificial colourings and flavourings.

In addition to eating different foods we are also eating less than we did 30 years ago because we are less physically active. But we still need the same amount of vitamins and minerals as we always have done. Because we eat less there's less chance of getting all those vital nutrients. You need to make sure that everything you eat is going to contribute actively towards your health.

The ingredients of a healthy diet

The basic principles of healthy eating are to choose your foods from four main food groups:

1 starchy foods – particularly wholegrain breads, cereals, rice, potatoes, pasta
2 fruit and vegetables
3 lean meat, including poultry, fish, nuts and pulses (peas and beans)
4 lower fat dairy products.

Figure 5 is a guide to getting the balance of foods right in your diet.

Starchy foods
Cereals and starchy vegetables, such as potatoes, are good sources of energy, fibre, vitamins and minerals.

Ideally you should eat 5 to 11 portions of these foods each day according to your appetite and your levels of activity. One portion is the equivalent of:

- an egg-sized potato
- one slice of bread/toast
- one wholewheat cereal biscuit
- three tablespoons of wholewheat breakfast cereal, eg branflakes
- three crackers or crispbreads
- one tablespoon of cooked rice, pasta or noodles

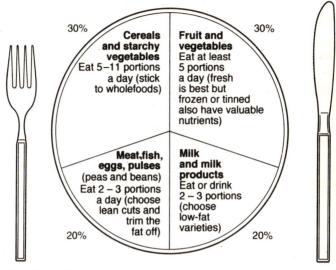

Fig. 5 The healthy balanced plate

Fruit and vegetables

Fruit and vegetables are high on the list of vital foods because it is known that the vitamins, minerals and fibre they contain can protect against heart disease, cancer and all sorts of other conditions.

A minimum of five portions a day is now recommended by the World Health Organization. A portion is classed as:

● one medium piece of fruit
● one medium carrot or tomato
● two tablespoons of vegetable (cooked or raw)
● two tablespoons tinned fruit in *natural juice*

Meat and fish

Meat, including poultry, and fish and their vegetarian alternatives, such as eggs, pulses and nuts, are good sources of protein. You should include two to three portions of these foods each day. A portion is:

- 2–4 oz (50–100g) lean meat or oily fish (like mackerel or salmon)
- 4–6 oz (100–175g) of white fish
- one or two eggs
- three tablespoons of cooked peas, beans or lentils
- two tablespoons of nuts or peanut butter (although as these foods tend to be high in fat they should be restricted)

Beware of over-indulging in protein foods. Research by Premsoc, the British-based charity researching PMS, has found that too much protein can block the absorption of nutrients such as vitamin B6, niacin, calcium, iron, zinc and magnesium. Since shortages of these vitamins and minerals have been implicated in PMS it is wise to stick to the recommended protein intakes.

Dairy products
Dairy products are an important source of calcium in our diets. If you are not eating any dairy products then you risk long-term problems of weak and brittle bones.

Other foods, such as green leafy vegetables, dried fruits and wholemeal bread, do contain calcium but in much lower levels than dairy products. For example you would have to eat nearly 1½lb (600g) of broccoli to obtain the same amount of calcium as in a 5oz (140g) pot of yoghurt.

Many women regard milk and dairy products as fattening but if you choose reduced-fat varieties you will still obtain all the good nutrients such as calcium and vitamin D without eating too much fat.

If you are still not convinced by the benefits of dairy foods then you should consider taking a daily calcium supplement to provide your body with this vital mineral.

At least two to three portions of milk and milk products should be included in your diet each day. A portion is:

- ⅓ pint (200ml) of milk
- a small tub of yoghurt
- 1 oz (30g) (about the size of a small matchbox) of hard cheese
- a small tub of cottage cheese

As you have probably noticed already there is a major omission from this list of foods. Yes, all those 'nice' things like cakes, chocolate, biscuits, croissants, pies, pastries, crisps are not on the list of healthy foods. These are the very foods which contain 'hidden' sugars and fats and should be avoided.

Other ingredients

Sugar

Sugar is considered by nutritional experts to be a 'non-essential' food. This means that we can do perfectly well without it.

Sugar is not bad in itself as it does provide the body with calories, but that is all. There are no vitamins or minerals in sugar so we would be far better off eating foods with natural sugar such as fruit and vegetables rather than filling up with sweets and cakes.

Of course sugar is fine on occasions but it should not be a staple part of the diet. Look out, too, for hidden sugars in soft drinks. Some cans of drink contain five teaspoons of sugar each!

PMS sufferers often crave sugary foods and it can be hard to resist those cravings. But if you are eating a healthy well-balanced diet, and you follow the advice given later in this chapter on eating little and often, you should be able to overcome, or at least reduce, those cravings.

Fats

We need small amounts of fat in our diet but most of us eat too much fat and what's more we eat the wrong kind of fat. Western diets are high in the saturated fats that have been linked to heart disease and other illnesses. If you choose your foods from the four groups listed and in the amounts given you will be getting all the fat you need from your diet.

Reducing fat in your diet

Since most people want to use fat for cooking or for spreading on bread, it is worth following these tips to try and reduce your fat intake:

- Avoid using butter or margarine on bread. If you do use it, choose a low fat variety and spread it very thinly.
- Use oils rather than solid fats when cooking. Measure cooking oils and salad oils carefully with a spoon rather than guessing the amount to use.
- Grill, steam or poach foods instead of frying.
- Do not add butter to cooked vegetables.

Salt

Salt is vital to our normal body function but as with sugar and fat the Western diet contains far too much for our needs.

The main problem for women with PMS is that salt attracts water, as anyone who has left their table salt in a damp room will know. In the body excess salt leads to water retention and the familiar PMS symptoms of bloating and puffiness.

A balanced diet will contain enough salt for all the body's needs so there is no need to add more during cooking or at the table.

Coffee and tea

Coffee and tea contain caffeine which is a natural diuretic – it encourages the kidneys to excrete more water in the urine.

In fact coffee and tea are a bit of a mixed blessing. They do relieve the symptoms of water retention but because caffeine is a stimulant it can exacerbate symptoms of anxiety and irritability and can prevent you relaxing and sleeping properly.

Most PMS doctors would advise cutting tea and coffee to no more than three or four cups a day. If you have trouble sleeping at night then try not to drink tea or coffee after 6pm as it takes roughly four hours for the caffeine to work through your system.

Also watch out for soft drinks as many of them contain caffeine.

Alcohol

Alcohol is not banned if you're a PMS sufferer but you do have to be careful.

Alcoholic drinks contain a lot of sugar which can play havoc with blood sugar levels. Many women with PMS find that they get drunk more easily when they are premenstrual. So be warned!

It is probably sensible to stick to the current recommended guidelines of a maximum of 14 units a week (1 unit = 1 glass of wine or 2 glasses of low alcohol wine, 1 measure of spirits, or ½ a pint of beer or lager).

Drinking one or two glasses each day is far better for you than blowing your alcohol limit at one heavy drinking session.

Combating PMS is not as simple as just eating the right foods. *When* you eat those foods has been shown to have a major influence on the symptoms of PMS also.

The PMS three-hourly starch diet

All the PMS self-help groups, and the majority of PMS specialist doctors, now recommend that women follow the PMS three-hourly starch diet.

The idea of the diet is to prevent blood sugar levels from dipping to the level where the body needs to release adrenalin. As discussed in Chapter 3, the body's attempts to maintain a steady blood sugar level by releasing adrenalin are thought to be at the root of many PMS symptoms.

According to Dr Maureen Dalton, of Sunderland Hospital in the UK, modern eating habits with large gaps between proper meals play havoc with our blood sugar levels.

'In the past women spent much of their time preparing food and while they were cooking they were also constantly nibbling which would have kept blood sugar at normal levels,' she says. 'It was also the custom to eat a large breakfast, have "elevenses", then lunch, tea, and dinner in the evening. There was no chance for blood sugar to go down'.

To understand this diet you need to know more about the different types of starchy foods – or *carbohydrates* – we eat.

More about carbohydrates

There are two types of carbohydrates – complex and simple:

Complex carbohydrates These are foods such as wholemeal bread, brown rice, wholegrain breakfast cereals, oats, potato, rye. They tend to be cereals in their natural state before processing. These foods take quite a long time for the body to break down into glucose – which is the form of energy the body needs – so they provide us with a steady flow of glucose over several hours. This helps to iron out any highs and lows of blood sugar.

Simple carbohydrates These include the refined foods such as white flour, sugar, honey, sweets, cakes, biscuits, white rice. They are very quickly digested by the body so they produce a rush of sugar into the bloodstream. To respond to this rush the body produces a large amount of insulin – a hormone that helps the liver to store the excess sugar from the blood.

Insulin quickly lowers the blood sugar. But often too much insulin is produced which means that too much sugar is taken out of the blood. Instead of going back to normal after eating a sugary snack the blood sugar will actually end up lower than before. So then the body is forced to produce adrenalin to get back some of the sugar from the liver and bring the blood sugar level back to normal.

Often you will feel the urge to eat some more sugary food to help the blood sugar back to normal. Then you are caught in a vicious circle of eating sugary food, feeling irritable and headachy because your blood sugar has dropped, eating more sugary food, feeling irritable and so on.

How to break the vicious circle

You need to steer clear of simple, refined sugars and starches. Women with PMS rarely have dangerously low blood sugar levels like those experienced by people being treated for diabetes.

Several studies have tested women given a sugary drink containing 2½oz (75g) of sugar. Four hours later, as their blood sugar dropped below normal, the women experienced sweating, palpitations, anxiety attacks, headaches and cravings for sweet food.

To avoid these symptoms you need to eat some sort of complex carbohydrate food every three hours during the day. The best foods to eat are those made with:

- wholemeal flour
- brown rice
- oats
- potato
- rye

If you're worried about putting on weight then be reassured that the three-hourly starch diet (*see* box 'The PMS three-hourly starch diet') does not mean eating more food. The aim is to spread your food intake more evenly throughout the day so instead of eating two or three meals you should eat six or seven times.

Crispbreads are an ideal low calorie complex carbohydrate food. Two crispbreads provide enough carbohydrate to keep you going for three hours and are only 30 calories – hardly fattening!

Does the three-hourly starch diet really work?

Dr Katharina Dalton has studied the three-hourly starch diet extensively at her London clinic. In one study she surveyed 84 women waiting for an appointment at the clinic and found that the average interval between eating carbohydrate during the day was seven hours, and overnight the average was 13.5 hours.

The women were asked to try the diet before their first appointment. As many as 70 per cent of the women reported an improvement in their symptoms after adhering to the three-hourly starch diet. The encouraging thing was that 23 per cent of the women with severe PMS managed to control their symptoms by adhering to the diet alone and without any further medical intervention.

The PMS three-hourly starch diet

Breakfast (always eaten within half an hour of getting up)
- five tablespoons cereal with low-fat milk or yoghurt
- a slice of wholemeal toast or bread with low-fat spread
- reduced-sugar marmalade or jam
- glass of fruit juice

Mid-morning snack
- one or two crispbreads *or*
- a small slice of wholemeal toast *or*
- a wholegrain digestive biscuit

Lunch
- a small jacket potato with cottage cheese and salad *or*
- half a sandwich, fruit and yoghurt

Mid-afternoon snack
- the other half of the sandwich *or*
- two crispbreads *or*
- a small slice of cake (made with wholewheat flour)

Supper
- lean meat or fish with vegetables or salad and potato or rice or pasta, followed by fruit or yoghurt or ice-cream *or*
- salad followed by fruit pie or cheesecake

Bedtime or late evening snack
- two crispbreads or crackers with a small cup of warm milk *or*
- a slice of bread with a small cup of warm milk

Drinks throughout the day
No more than four cups of coffee or tea (ideally decaffeinated) with plenty of plain water and no more than two glasses of fruit juice taken with meals.

This menu is only a guide. The important thing to remember is that complex carbohydrates should be eaten regularly throughout the day.

Exercise

Fitness levels in the Western world as a whole have declined dramatically in the last 30 years. Today we go everywhere by car. We sit at our desks for long hours. We slump in front of the television night after night. As with healthy eating it only takes a little effort to break the couch-potato cycle. There are several benefits to be gained from taking exercise:

- It increases your levels of fitness and helps you to combat illness. Lack of exercise leads to increased weight gain, weak muscles, weak bones and a sluggish heart. Although lack of exercise is not exactly a cause of PMS, more activity will improve your general health.
- Exercise has been shown to increase levels of endorphins in the brain. Endorphins are often referred to as the body's natural 'happy' chemicals as they help to lift our mood and ease pain. Several studies have shown that people who are depressed show a significant improvement in their symptoms if they take regular exercise.
- Taking regular exercise improves your self-esteem and makes you feel good about yourself. In this frame of mind you are much better equipped to cope with PMS than the couch-potato whose idea of physical activity is going to the kitchen to fetch a snack!

Taking more exercise does not mean buying the latest trendy aerobic gear and enrolling at the local health club.

The simplest exercise regime is to walk. A practical exercise regime for most women is to walk for three miles (5km) or 45 minutes (whichever comes first: one mile (1½km) every 15 minutes is ideal). Do this at least three or four times a week. Once this is comfortable you can increase the rate to one mile every 10 to 12 minutes.

Jogging, cycling, swimming or aerobic exercise are great if you can fit them into your schedule and you do them for at least 30 minutes three times a week.

Many women are restricted by the demands of a family. But children benefit from walking too so take them with you. If you have a baby put it in the buggy or the baby sling and get out there!

Give it time

Don't expect overnight results from changing your diet and taking more exercise. If you've spent a lifetime eating junk and sitting around all day it's going to take several months to undo the damage.

You should start seeing an improvement after two months. But don't be tempted to slink back to your old habits. After all those old habits are what got you into this mess in the first place so stick at it!

CHAPTER 5

Stress and PMS

How to reduce stress and relieve your PMS

Stress is so important in PMS that it warrants this whole chapter of its own. The research just emerging shows that PMS and stress go hand-in-hand. If you have a lot of stress in your life you are more likely to develop PMS. Women with PMS often have more stress in their lives than women without the condition, according to Dr Jane Chihal from Texas, USA.

'Perhaps stress predisposes the patient to PMS or perhaps the syndrome can be perceived as a type of inner stress. If a patient also experiences external stress, the total stress "load" may exacerbate the severity of her symptoms,' she says.

Professor Shaughn O'Brien of Keele University in the UK agrees. Although he runs a 'conventional' PMS clinic he advocates the use of relaxation and stress management techniques to help relieve PMS.

What is stress?

Stress is something that we generate inside ourselves in response to 'stressors'. Stressors can be major events such as crumbling relationships, a dead-end job or delinquent children – but they can also be simply the accumulating daily hassles of constant deadlines and snatched meals. In other words, they can be anything that leads to stress.

In fact not all stressors are nasty. Winning the lottery, or going on holiday can trigger as much of a stress response as having your handbag snatched on the way to work.

Intense emotion such as excitement, anxiety, frustration and anger is the trigger for the body's stress reaction.

In primitive times the stress response was a vital part of our defence against danger such as being chased by wild animals. The stress response makes us ready for immediate physical action whether running as fast as we can to escape or stopping to fight. This is known as 'the fight or flight response'.

The body responds to a stressor in several ways (*see* Figure 6):

- adrenalin and glucose flood into the body
- breathing becomes shallow and fast to take in more oxygen
- muscles contract ready for use
- blood pressure increases
- the heart beats faster

Stress can feel good. Adrenalin can give you a buzz and almost make you feel 'high'. This is fine when you are racing to meet a deadline, for example, and you need that extra burst of energy to rise to the challenge.

But stress becomes bad when the chemicals released during the stress reaction stay in the body. In prehistoric times the stress reaction would always have been followed by a burst of physical activity which would have broken down the chemicals allowing the body to relax afterwards.

In modern times it appears that often the chemicals produced by the stress reaction are not broken down before we meet another stressor which starts the whole process again. This means our bodies never return to normal and we are in a permanent state of stress.

Typical signs of built-up stress

- inability to sleep properly
- unexplained aches and pains
- indigestion
- feeling tired all the time
- a feeling of having too much to do and too little time to do it
- uncontrolled eating
- chain smoking
- drinking too much alcohol
- lack of interest in sex
- crying for no reason
- outbursts of temper
- sweating/palpitations
- shortness of breath and/or dizziness
- feeling tired as soon as you wake up
- twitching muscles, especially the eyes

If you recognize several of these signs in yourself then the alarm bells should be ringing. You could be under too much stress.

For many of us the image of a stressed-out individual is a middle-aged company executive who works all hours, eats too many heavy business lunches, smokes like a chimney and is well on his way to his first coronary. But women are not immune to stress.

In fact the dual pressures of home and work are putting women under extraordinary levels of stress. A recent survey of 20,000 British men and women found that 42 per cent of the women reported being under stress compared with 30 per cent of the men. Women today, it seems, may be more stressed than men.

In the UK women now make up more than half the workforce but are still responsible for 80 per cent of the country's housework, in addition to taking most of the burden of caring for children. And it's not just working women who are under stress.

Studies of stay-at-home mothers have consistently found that they are more depressed and have lower self-esteem than their working counterparts.

What has stress got to do with PMS?

Looking through the list of stress symptoms there are some obvious similarities with PMS. In fact studies in the USA by Dr Irene Goodale, of Harvard University medical school, have shown that in the luteal phase of their menstrual cycle women have a higher than normal response to stress compared with the rest of the time:

- their heart rate goes up
- blood pressure increases
- more adrenalin is released
- urine samples have higher levels of adrenalin and noradrenalin – both signs of stress.

If you have PMS and you are under a lot of stress your body will be under a double dose of pressure. It's important that in seeking a cure for your PMS you do not ignore the influence of stress. There is simply no point in treating your PMS if your stress is out of control. You will either not respond to PMS therapy or those symptoms will clear up and you will succumb to something else.

In dealing with stress you can either avoid the stressors or you can learn to cope with the stress. In practice it's impossible to avoid all stressors so it's best to develop coping strategies.

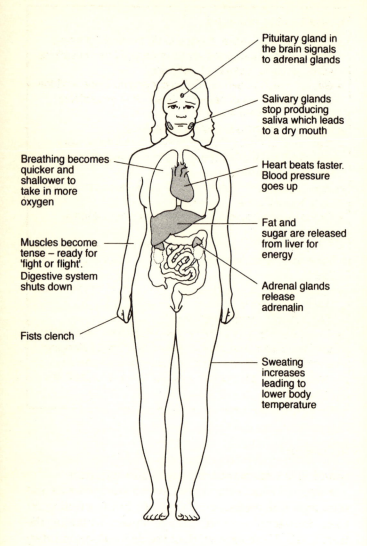

Fig. 6 The effects of stress on the body

Stress-busting strategies

- Take regular exercise. It helps to rid the body of stress chemicals and increases levels of natural brain chemicals which promote a sense of wellbeing.
- Get out into the open air. Being cooped up indoors all the time deprives you of natural light which is essential to help maintain your mood.
- Allow yourself time to get plenty of sleep.
- Simplify your life by cutting down on technology; ask yourself if you really need a mobile phone or a fax machine at home.
- Rediscover nature. Watch insects or birds go about their daily business – it's very relaxing.
- Go home from work earlier. Long hours do not mean greater efficiency.
- Delegate responsibility. If the children have never washed the dishes or cleaned up their rooms it's time for them to learn.
- Allow more time to get to appointments so that you're not always in a hurry.
- Take all your holiday entitlement.
- Take up a hobby or sport or join in more with community affairs and discover a sense of self-worth and belonging.
- Don't succumb to road rage. If someone cuts you up in traffic simply carry on with your journey and forget it. It's their problem.

Relaxation

Learning to relax is the best way of tackling stress.

Have you ever been on holiday to a warm climate and seen the local people simply sitting in the evening on their doorsteps or in the village square watching the world go by? The hard work of the day is done and they are content to simply relax and take it easy.

Most people in the industrialized world have forgotten how to relax like that. We are so busy rushing around trying to 'get things done' that we never have time to stop and think about why we're behaving in this crazy way.

Taking time to relax is as important as eating a good diet and taking regular exercise. But it is not just a case of taking time out to do nothing. Like everything, you have to work at relaxation if you're not used to it.

There's no point doing nothing for half an hour if your mind is still buzzing with the day's events, money worries, children's problems, what you're going to cook for dinner. To relax fully you need to use the time to get in touch with your mind and emotions.

There are lots of ways of relaxing. Taking a warm bath, sitting in the evening sun with a cool drink, taking a stroll round the park, can all be effective. Or you may prefer a more structured approach – meditation or yoga, perhaps. Whatever way you choose there is evidence that relaxation can significantly reduce PMS symptoms.

Dr Goodale's work at Harvard has shown significant reductions in PMS in women who are taught how to relax. She studied 46 women who were put into three groups. Group one were asked to simply record their symptoms every day. Group two were told to record their symptoms and to read a book for at least 30 minutes each day. Group three were taught a relaxation technique which involved clearing the mind and focusing on a repetitive mental activity such as counting.

The three groups did this for at least 20 minutes each day and at the end of the three-month study the relaxation group showed a significantly greater improvement in their physical and psychological PMS symptoms compared with the other groups.

But reading was not a total waste of time as this group improved significantly compared with the group that simply recorded symptoms.

The exciting thing was that women with the most severe symptoms benefited the most with a 58 per cent improvement in the relaxation group, compared with 27.2 per cent in the reading group and 17 per cent in group one.

Dr Goodale admits that the study did not answer the question of how relaxation can relieve PMS. But she believes that the body is increasingly sensitive to adrenalin in the days before a period which explains the increased aggression and anxiety associated with PMS. Relaxation reduces this sensitivity and in doing so helps to relieve symptoms.

The key is that relaxation is a proven way of reducing PMS. So if you haven't tried it now is the time to start.

Clare's story

'I was the typical '90s superwoman or thought I was,' says Clare, 39, who runs a public relations business near Bristol in western Britain. 'I'd spent years building up my business and we'd got to the stage where things were doing well. I had four staff and a good portfolio of clients. So I decided to have a baby.

'I went back to work when Gemma was six weeks old because I felt I couldn't leave the business any longer. From then on things went downhill.

'I was working really long hours. My diet was terrible because I didn't have the energy to cook properly in the evenings. On top of that I hardly ever had a good night's sleep because Gemma was very unsettled at night.

'PMS sort of crept up on me. I felt exhausted, which I thought was due to Gemma. I was so snappy and bad-tempered that I must have been impossible to live with. Nothing anyone did was right. I also used to get such a bloated abdomen that I couldn't do up my skirt buttons.

'My family doctor was really sympathetic. She inspired me to change my diet and to sort out my life so that I wasn't putting in so many hours at work and at home. She said I needed to take time for myself so I joined a yoga class at my local health club.

'It took quite a while for things to start improving. But I realized that I'd been heading towards a breakdown and PMS was just a warning signal. Now I take a much more relaxed approach to things and I actually think that I am more effective at work because of it.

'My PMS has not totally disappeared but it's manageable and it doesn't cause the chaos it used to'.

CHAPTER 6

Conventional treatments and procedures

What your doctor will probably say and do

There's no simple treatment for PMS so doctors generally do find it hard to treat. What works for one woman may not work for another, even though their symptoms are identical.

The good news is that conventionally-trained doctors are much more likely to regard PMS as a serious condition than they were 10 or 15 years ago.

But few family doctors have the time or resources to treat PMS properly. As we have seen from the previous chapters, PMS treatment starts with changes to diet, exercise and stress. In the UK the average consultation with a family doctor is under 10 minutes – hardly time to listen to the patient's symptoms let alone explore self-help issues. There are a few enlightened doctors who have set up PMS clinics where women have time to talk through their problems. Sadly, though, these are rare. But it's still worth asking if your family doctor runs one or can refer you to one.

When you do see your doctor don't be surprised if he or she is sceptical about your self-diagnosis of PMS. Studies in the USA and the UK have shown that up to 50 per cent of women who believe they have PMS do not have it. Often they have another problem such as clinical depression which they mistake for PMS. Be prepared for this scepticism by taking in your diary of symptoms.

What your doctor *should* say and do

The doctor should ask plenty of questions. You should be asked about:

- Symptoms you experience, their severity and how long they last. You may be asked whether PMS seriously affects your life or if it is merely an inconvenience. If you have not already done so you should be asked to complete a diary of symptoms.
- Menstrual pattern. How regular are your periods? Do you have other problems such as menstrual cramps, abnormally heavy bleeding?
- Contraceptive needs. One of the treatments used in PMS is the oral contraceptive pill and if this fits in with what you want to use as a contraceptive then this may be the first treatment the doctor will prescribe.
- Childbirth. Did PMS start after a pregnancy? Did you have postnatal depression?
- Self-help measures. What have you tried and what were the results?
- Other physical symptoms. You may be given an internal examination. If you report physical symptoms such as breast pain or abdominal bloating the doctor should want to exclude another possible cause for the symptoms.

A blood sample should be taken to test for low levels of iron (*anaemia*), thyroid disorders, and even the menopause – all of which can be mistaken for PMS.

If you are one of the women who experiences hot flushes premenstrually then your doctor will be keen to find out whether you are approaching the menopause. Women in their mid- to late-40s often experience menopausal symptoms such as hot flushes and pain on sexual intercourse long before their periods stop.

If you are in this age group you will have a blood

sample taken to check for levels of follicle-stimulating hormone. Even if you are not in this age group up to 1 per cent of women have their menopause before the age of 40 so do not be surprised if your doctor checks for the possibility of premature menopause.

You may be surprised at the questions your doctor asks, particularly those about your mood, family circumstances, and stress. The doctor is asking these questions to help him or her distinguish between *primary* PMS and *secondary* PMS.

- Primary PMS is 'pure' PMS – the symptoms you describe only occur premenstrually and are completely absent after the start of menstruation.
- Secondary PMS is PMS which occurs in addition to an underlying psychological or psychiatric condition such as depression or anxiety.

Sometimes doctors have trouble diagnosing PMS. In this case you may be offered a three-month trial of a drug, such as the oral contraceptive pill, which blocks the normal menstrual cycle. If, after three to six months, you are still experiencing the same symptoms it is highly likely that the problem is not PMS.

Medical treatment of PMS

Doctors usually start with a treatment that will have the fewest side-effects. If it works, good. If not, then something else will have to be tried. Figure 7 (on page 53) shows a typical approach to managing PMS.

Vitamin B6 (pyridoxine)

This is one of the oldest PMS therapies and dates from the discovery that B6 is involved in the production of serotonin and dopamine, two of the 'happy' chemicals in the brain.

The current therapy is 100mg a day taken by mouth. The treatment is taken for the whole month, not just when you are likely to be premenstrual.

But the evidence for vitamin B6's efficacy is shaky. An analysis of 12 clinical trials of vitamin B6 found three with positive results, five with ambiguous results and four with negative results. Dutch researchers who analysed the B6 trials said: 'At the moment there is no evidence that vitamin B6 is efficacious in the treatment of patients with PMS'.

Despite this, some women do seem to improve when they are taking vitamin B6 and for this reason many doctors are prepared to give it a try.

High doses of vitamin B6 are known to cause nerve damage resulting in symptoms like pins and needles, muscle weakness and even eye damage. The general consensus is that 100mg a day is unlikely to cause problems and it is well worth sticking to that dose if you have been prescribed this medicine.

Evening primrose oil

Evening primrose oil is widely available through health-food shops, pharmacists and, in the UK, can be obtained on prescription for the treatment of breast pain (*mastalgia*). It is not available on prescription for the treatment of PMS but if you have cyclical breast pain your doctor may consider prescribing it.

Although it is effective at treating breast pain, the evidence for its effect on other PMS symptoms is not so clear. A recent article in the *British Medical Journal* said that, while questions remain about how evening primrose oil should be used, it was an 'interesting substance' and 'showed promise' in the treatment of PMS. So it's worth trying.

The recommended level for treatment of breast pain is

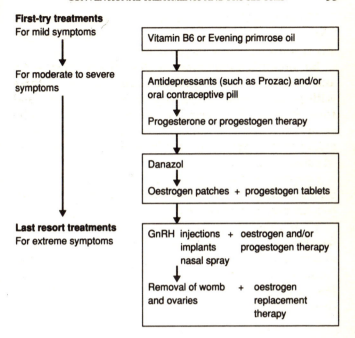

First-try treatments
For mild symptoms

For moderate to severe
symptoms

Last resort treatments
For extreme symptoms

Vitamin B6 or Evening primrose oil

Antidepressants (such as Prozac) and/or
oral contraceptive pill

Progesterone or progestogen therapy

Danazol

Oestrogen patches + progestogen tablets

GnRH injections + oestrogen and/or
         implants   progestogen therapy
         nasal spray

Removal of womb + oestrogen
and ovaries   replacement
                         therapy

Fig. 7 Medical and surgical treatments for PMS

three to four 'prescription dose' capsules, taken twice a
day. The prescription dose is 40mg of *gamma-linolenic-
acid* (GLA), the main active ingredient in evening primrose oil. But don't expect instant results. It can take up to
three months to see any improvement. The usual course
of treatment is six to twelve months, although some
women find it helpful to carry on.

If you are buying evening primrose oil for self-treat-
ment it is important to buy capsules with the right dose
for your needs. Capsules sold in the shops usually contain 250mg or 500mg of evening primrose oil but only
the 500mg preparation contains 40mg of GLA so make
sure you check the label.

You will need to take two or three 500mg capsules twice daily after food. It is usually recommended that you start taking the capsules from three days before the expected start of your symptoms until your period is fully under way. But if you have erratic cycles, or have had a hysterectomy, or your symptoms are very severe, then you may be advised to take the capsules right through the month.

Diuretics

Diuretics are a standard treatment for water retention and will be of no help for other PMS symptoms. They work by interfering with normal kidney function so that the kidneys excrete more urine.

PMS specialists tend to agree that diuretics should be reserved for women who actually gain weight in the luteal phase of the menstrual cycle. Some women develop abdominal bloating but do not put on weight and it is questionable whether they are retaining water at all or simply that their weight is redistributed just before a period. If you are not retaining water then a diuretic should *not* be prescribed.

There are problems with diuretics as they can cause even worse water retention – rebound water retention – when you stop taking them. Some diuretics may cause a deficiency of the mineral *potassium* leading to symptoms of weakness and confusion and, in severe cases, heart palpitations.

The diuretic most often prescribed for PMS is *spironolactone* which is thought to carry a lower risk of rebound water retention.

Antidepressants and tranquillizers

The discovery that women with PMS have low serotonin levels in the brain has led doctors to try drugs which raise serotonin. These drugs are known collectively as antidepressants. The best known is Prozac (chemical name *fluoxetine*).

One of the first studies of Prozac in PMS looked at 21 women with premenstrual depression. They took Prozac or a dummy pill for three months. After that they swapped treatments. None of the women, or the doctors treating them, knew which drugs each woman was taking until after the study had finished.

There was a striking reduction in symptoms in the women taking Prozac compared with those on placebo. Symptoms quickly returned in the majority of women once the Prozac therapy had ended.

The New Zealand researchers who conducted the study said that the work had supported the theory that PMS was in part caused by low serotonin in the brain as well as showing that this drug could be effective in treating severe PMS.

The current recommended dose of Prozac is 20mg a day by mouth and most doctors would restrict it to women who had severe psychological symptoms, such as depression, as part of their PMS.

Tranquillizers – drugs that treat anxiety – are rarely used for PMS nowadays as it is recognized that they can be addictive. One of the best known examples is Valium. They often cause more problems than they solve and would only be prescribed for a very short time – days rather than weeks.

Oral contraceptive pill

'The Pill' – usually a combination of oestrogen and a synthetic type of progesterone – is a common treatment for PMS because it suppresses the normal menstrual cycle. Some women experience complete relief from their symptoms and it can be quite a shock to the system if you've come off the Pill after several years and are hit with all your old symptoms again.

For a minority of women the Pill can trigger depression. Sometimes vitamin B6 will be prescribed to treat pill-associated depression but if that does not work then a change in the type of progestogen in the pill may be needed.

Progesterone/progestogen therapy

Progesterone therapy is one of the most controversial therapies for PMS, yet it is one of the most widely used. Supporters of British researcher Dr Katharina Dalton, who has researched the treatment for over 30 years, are largely responsible for its widespread use.

Despite the enthusiasm, proper studies of progesterone versus a dummy pill have failed to show any benefit with this hormone therapy. But because a few women do seem to benefit many doctors feel it's worth a try if other methods have failed.

Dr Dalton and other doctors who follow her teaching believe that natural progesterone should not be taken by mouth because it breaks down before it has a chance to work. So vaginal or rectal 'suppositories' – a gel-based 'pellet' inserted into the vagina or rectum – are used instead. Sometimes daily injections are given and work is being done on a tablet form.

The dose is 400mg to 800mg taken twice a day, starting on day 12 of the cycle. Treatment usually lasts for a minimum of six months but some women may need to carry on for up to two years or until the menopause if they are over 40.

Progestogens are synthetic forms of progesterone which can be taken as tablets by mouth.

Dydrogesterone is the type of progestogen most often prescribed. The main drawback of progestogens is that some women find they tend to produce more side-effects than natural progesterone, especially weight gain and irregular periods.

Critics of progestogen treatment say its chemical structure is so different from that of progesterone that it does not work and actually makes PMS worse. Once again, though, there have been no studies to support or refute this claim.

Oestrogen therapy

Oestrogen is prescribed on the basis that PMS occurs at the time of the cycle when natural oestrogen is at its lowest. So what is needed is to keep oestrogen high for the whole month – blocking the natural menstrual cycle in the process.

The most common way of taking oestrogen is in a patch stuck on to the skin or an implant underneath the skin. Implants are replaced every six months while patches are changed every three days.

The main drawback is that oestrogen causes a buildup of the lining of the womb and this increases the risk of *endometrial cancer* (cancer of the womb). To ensure that the womb lining is shed regularly, a one-week course of progestogen tablets has to be taken every month. Some women find this brings back their PMS although it is often easier to cope with as the symptoms are not so severe.

Some studies of oestrogen patches have found that PMS symptoms get worse before they get better so if you are prescribed this therapy you will be warned to per-severe with treatment for at least a month.

Critics have said that oestrogen patches and implants are no different from taking the contraceptive pill. But with the Pill the progestogen is taken every day of the month whereas with implants or patches it is taken for only seven days which reduces the symptoms.

Bromocriptine

Bromocriptine is a drug that blocks the production of the hormone *prolactin*, which is thought to trigger premenstrual breast symptoms. It is prescribed as a 2.5mg tablet to be taken at night.

Danazol

Danazol is a drug related to the 'male' hormone testoterone. It is used for a number of gynaecological conditions including endometriosis, heavy periods and some breast diseases.

It is generally reserved for severe cases of PMS and works by suppressing ovulation and menstruation. But danazol has some significant side-effects including weight gain, nausea, giddiness.

In addition danazol has a masculinizing effect so some women experience acne, grow facial hair and find that their breasts decrease in size. In the long term danazol can also affect blood cholesterol levels so it is usually taken for no more than six months.

Gonadotrophin-releasing hormone (GnRH) analogues

These drugs are used for the most severe cases and work by blocking the pituitary hormones that trigger the menstrual cycle. In effect they produce a sort of minimenopause because no oestrogen is produced by the body.

To prevent long-term problems caused by lack of oestrogen – such as weak bones and raised cholesterol levels – oestrogen therapy is usually prescribed at the same time.

GnRH analogues are given as a nasal spray or long-acting injection.

Doctors who use this therapy say it can be invaluable in women whose marriages are deteriorating as a direct result of PMS as it can give a break from symptoms. The other advantage is that the break from symptoms shows the woman and her family that there is a biological explanation for the symptoms and that they are not due to psychiatric or personality disorders.

Surgery

Surgery (hysterectomy) is an extremely rare treatment for PMS and not one to be taken lightly. It involves removing the womb and the ovaries, resulting in instant menopause. Oestrogen replacement therapy is needed for life after this type of surgery.

It should only be considered as a last-ditch attempt at solving really serious PMS.

Hysterectomy is a major step so if your doctor refers you to a surgeon who offers this option you should take time to think and discuss the implications with your partner. If you are not sure, it is definitely worth getting a second opinion from another doctor before agreeing to anything.

CHAPTER 7

The natural therapies and PMS

Introducing the gentle alternatives

Doctors admit that they do not have all the answers to PMS. Some of their medications work and others don't – and often they don't know why. Many women, disillusioned with what conventional medicine has to offer, are turning to natural therapies in their quest for relief from distressing symptoms.

There seem to be three main reasons for this:

- Some women feel that medications that completely suppress the menstrual cycle are a rather drastic measure to take when all they want is relief from PMS.
- Since the long-term effects of some medicines are unknown, many women would prefer a treatment that is less likely to be harmful.
- Conventional doctors simply do not have the resources to deal with PMS. In the UK there are fewer than 20 clinics for PMS run by the free state-run National Health Service and these deal only with the most intractable cases. The majority of PMS patients are dealt with by family doctors who, with all their other commitments, usually find it hard to fit in full evaluation and treatment of PMS.

Who uses natural therapy?

The number of people visiting natural therapists is rocketing throughout the world. In Britain, for example, a recent survey by the Consumers' Association found that one in four of its members had visited a practitioner of natural medicine – nearly double the number who had tried natural therapy in a similar survey three years previously.

Conventional doctors themselves are also more willing to accept that natural therapies may have something to offer. The British Medical Association reported in 1994 that nearly three-quarters of British family doctors had referred a patient to a natural therapist at some time and that 80 per cent of trainee doctors wished to train in one or more of the natural therapies in addition to their conventional training.

Estimates of the number of doctors who practise natural therapies themselves range from 2 to 15 per cent. In the UK alone the number of medically-qualified doctors who also practise homoeopathy has risen from 200 to more than 1,000 in less than a decade. Although that is a tiny proportion of the 35,000 family doctors in the UK, the numbers are still rising. A course for family doctors in homoeopathy at Glasgow Homoeopathic Hospital in Scotland is Britain's most popular postgraduate medical course: one in ten Scottish family doctors has taken it.

But though it remains true that more doctors are taking up the practice of such natural therapies as, particularly, homoeopathy and acupuncture, most people will still have to seek out a specialist in the various natural therapies rather than a doctor for treatment this way.

Why go to a natural therapist?

Surveys of patients using natural practitioners have found there are two main reasons for turning to these forms of therapy.

The top reason is disappointing experiences with conventional doctors. A Dutch study found that 39 per cent of people using a natural therapist had been unhappy with the service they had received from conventional doctors.

The next most common reason is that a friend or relative has recommended the therapy.

Some people turn to natural (also known as 'complementary' or 'alternative') medicine as a last resort but only a small proportion of patients surveyed cited a firm belief in the natural therapy as their reason for going to a natural therapist.

Whatever their reasons for turning to natural therapy, most people seem to be very satisfied with the treatment they receive. In the UK, the Consumers' Association found that four out of five of its members who used a natural therapist claim to have been cured or have had their symptoms improved by a natural therapist – and three-quarters of them said they would visit a natural therapist again.

What is natural therapy?

On the surface it sometimes appears that the natural therapies have little in common. What has herbalism, using plants to heal, in common with reflexology, a system of healing through foot manipulation, for example? In fact, although the various therapies employ a wide range of techniques, they are all based on a similar approach to healing.

● Symptoms are assessed in relation to the personality of

the patient. First, a natural therapist will want to get an overall picture of the patient's personality so that treatment can be tailored to the individual. Unlike conventional medicine, the treatment administered by a natural therapist for a condition like PMS may vary from one woman to another depending on that woman's individual makeup and circumstances.

- The whole person is treated, not just the symptoms. The natural practitioner will break down barriers between mind and body so that the whole person can be healed. This will mean a full assessment of lifestyle, personality, stresses, state of mind and natural energy.
- Many therapies are based on the idea that illness occurs when the body's systems are out of balance and in a state of 'dis-ease' and therapy will aim to restore that balance.
- Natural therapists are not simply concerned with removing the immediate symptoms but will work to restore people to a state of health and wellbeing where they will be able to avoid further illness. They recognize that someone who has low resistance to infection and is in poor general health will need more than a quick-fix cure. Often a natural therapist will work with an individual long after the original symptoms have cleared up to help them achieve a higher state of physical and mental wellbeing.
- The goal of natural therapy is self-healing. Most of the therapies recognize that each individual has some power for self-healing that may need to be harnessed more effectively. This means that patients are encouraged to help themselves. If you are used to visiting a conventional doctor who simply writes out a prescription for your cure you may find that a natural therapist will expect more input from you. There is more of a partnership between patient and therapist towards the goal of maintaining good health.

What to expect when you see a natural therapist

The most striking difference between natural therapy and conventional medicine is the length of time you will spend in consultation with your therapist. A first consultation with a natural therapist is likely to take at least an hour and much of the time will be spent in finding out about you and your life. Further consultations are unlikely to be as long as the first but will still be longer than you would spend with a family doctor.

Treatments are different too. Often, after the initial symptoms have cleared, you will continue to receive some form of therapy aimed at restoring your body's natural healing ability. For this reason treatments may take longer than those used in conventional medicine. They may also take longer to work.

In addition to specific treatments you will usually be advised to make changes to your lifestyle – for example, a change of diet, sleeping habits, stress management, and exercise may all be recommended to help you back to good health.

You will not be a passive recipient of healthcare. A natural therapist will encourage you to take more responsibility for your own health.

Do the natural therapies work?

This is one of the most hotly-debated issues in medical circles. Natural practitioners are convinced of the benefits of their therapies but they have had a hard time convincing conventional doctors.

Though there are a lot of satisfied customers, that is no proof that natural therapies work. Doctors want hard proof, usually in the form of strictly-conducted clinical trials.

A clinical trial usually compares a medicine with a dummy pill in patients who do not know which pill they are taking. A dummy pill (known as a 'placebo') which is identical in appearance to the active drug is used because it is known that patients can show an improvement in their condition if they think they are receiving a cure. This is known as the 'placebo effect'. If the medicine is shown to be statistically more effective than the placebo then it can be said to work.

The problem with the natural therapies is that they are often not suited to the strict controls of clinical trials. Since practitioners may treat people differently according to their individual circumstances it is virtually impossible to compare like with like. Also, it is difficult in some of the therapies to have a placebo group: in acupuncture, for example, how do you give a 'dummy' needle?

There have been some attempts to prove that natural therapies work and to have the results of clinical trials published in reputable medical journals. One of the largest was an analysis of 107 clinical trials of homoeopathy carried out by a Dutch medical team and published in the *British Medical Journal*.

But the authors of the analysis concluded that most of the trials were of such poor quality that it was impossible to draw conclusions. Of the well-conducted studies 15 showed positive results, and in seven trials no positive result could be detected or the outcome was negative. They concluded that more research was needed.

Despite the lack of clinical research into the natural therapies there is some evidence that they are of benefit for conditions such as PMS. Treatments tend to fall into two groups: physical therapies and psychological therapies. But there is often quite a bit of overlap between the two. For PMS the therapies said to be beneficial include the following.

Psychological therapies
- Hypnosis/hypnotherapy
- Biofeedback
- Psychotherapy (including cognitive therapy and counselling)
- Meditation
- Autogenics
- Creative visualization
- Art/drama/horticultural therapy
- Yoga

Physical therapies
- Acupuncture
- Herbal medicine (Western and Oriental traditions)
- Nutritional medicine
- Homoeopathy
- Naturopathy
- Aromatherapy and massage
- Reflexology

Some of these therapies are backed by good research to support their use while others are used because natural therapists and their patients find them beneficial.

It can be quite daunting to choose a natural therapy if you have no knowledge of the principles on which they are based. The following two chapters outline the approaches taken by these therapies and Chapter 10 is a guide to finding and choosing a natural therapist you can rely on.

CHAPTER 8

Treating your mind and emotions

Psychological therapies for PMS

If you have read this far you will have learnt that the mind can have a considerable influence on physical symptoms and PMS is one of those conditions that is directly affected by emotional and psychological circumstances.

It's now clear that a healthy mind goes hand-in-hand with a healthy body. The psychological therapies may not necessarily cure PMS but they do relieve the stresses and strains that make PMS worse. Once these stresses are removed many women find that their PMS goes too – or at least that they now have the inner resources to cope.

Hypnosis/Hypnotherapy

If you've seen a stage hypnotist in action then you have probably got the wrong idea about hypnotherapy. A professional hypnotherapist will use hypnosis as part of an overall package of psychological therapy to help you overcome deep-seated barriers to full health. You won't walk out of their office and start stripping off in the street or make rude remarks to passers-by.

Hypnotherapy from a reputable practitioner will not make you do anything you don't want to because you will never lose total control of your actions. The aim of hypnotherapy is to put you into a suggestible state of mind or trance where you can readily accept suggestions from the therapist. They may suggest, for example, that you are gaining confidence, that you are overcoming your PMS, that you are not angry any more.

There has been little clinical research into hypnotherapy and PMS (though hypnotherapy as a whole is one of the best researched of the natural therapies) but it is well accepted by the medical profession as a useful treatment for conditions as diverse as irritable bowel syndrome, asthma and back pain. It is also used to help prepare patients for major surgery and to help reduce the side-effects of cancer chemotherapy.

In the USA, UK, Australia and most Western countries many large hospitals employ at least one member of staff trained in hypnotherapy, and many family doctors refer their patients for the treatment.

A course of hypnotherapy is likely to last 12 weeks, consisting of one session a week with each session lasting from 45 to 60 minutes.

To put you into a trance the therapist will talk to you slowly and in a relaxed manner. They may ask you to concentrate on an image such as a walk by the sea where the waves are pounding rhythmically on the beach. Or they may repeat a series of monotonous words, or colours.

Next you will be told your eyes are feeling heavy and are closing. At this stage you will be in a light trance. You may be put into a deeper trance by the therapist counting from one to ten or asking you to imagine going down in a lift.

At this stage the therapist might help you work out any deep-seated problems you may have or make suggestions for self-healing.

What the therapist will *not* do is promise to 'cure' you. Hypnotherapy can be immensely helpful in building up your confidence and helping you back to full health but it is not a cure. Therapists who advertise that they can cure PMS or that you can lose weight or quit cigarettes in one easy session are usually more interested in your money than your health and should be avoided.

This is one of the few natural therapies where you would be best advised to ask your family doctor or PMS specialist for a referral to a qualified hypnotherapist (but *see* Appendix A – Useful Organizations). The practice is generally not well regulated and levels of training and expertise vary widely.

Biofeedback

This is a 'hi-tech' way of teaching you how to relax. You will be fitted with equipment which records your pulse rate, or blood pressure, temperature, muscle tension, amount of sweat on your skin or even your brainwaves. The recordings are displayed on a screen in front of you.

You will then be taught to lower your readings by relaxation. Gradually over several sessions you will learn how to change your bodily functions – a sign that you are relaxing. Eventually you will no longer need a machine to help you. Biofeedback is widely used in migraine treatment so if you have premenstrual headaches this may help you.

Counselling and psychotherapy

'A problem shared is a problem halved' is an old saying and it's true. Often we feel a lot better when we've 'got things off our chest' and had a good talk with a friend.

Counselling is simply a formal way of providing someone to talk to but often it is more effective than just talking to a friend. A trained counsellor who is not involved in your life is able to provide a more detached, unbiased and honest way of listening.

The aim is to encourage you to talk about your feelings and problems. You will then discuss these with the counsellor and together will explore ways of understanding your problems. Counselling is not a medical therapy but it can help resolve issues that are making physical and psychological problems worse.

Psychotherapy is a more detailed form of counselling. The aim is to help patients learn about themselves, their past and present relationships and teach them how to change fixed patterns of behaviour.

It's worth pointing out that a psychotherapist, even a well-trained one, is not a doctor and is not allowed to prescribe drug treatments. A medical doctor trained in dealing with mental disorders, usually with drugs, is called a *psychiatrist*.

One of the most successful psychotherapies used in PMS is 'cognitive therapy'. Cognitive therapy is based on the idea that the way we think about ourselves and others influences our emotions and behaviour.

For example, someone who is depressed may believe that everything bad that happens to them is their own fault and that anything good is just luck.

If they are walking along the road and they shout 'hello' to a friend and the friend ignores them the depressed person will believe the friend no longer likes them or wants to talk to them. They may brood on the incident for the rest of the day. Another person who is not depressed will realize that the friend had not heard them and will shout louder next time.

A cognitive therapist will help the patient recognize a negative attitude to life which is preventing them from being well. They will help them develop a more positive outlook and explore various behavioural changes that the patient can make – like being more self-assertive, or talking with their husband or partner about sharing household chores or childcare.

A course of cognitive therapy usually takes about 12 weekly sessions. Studies of people with mild to moderate depression have shown that it is as effective as medication, although it may take longer to show results. Pilot studies of a very small number of women taking part in several large-scale studies of PMS under way in 1995 had shown improvements in wellbeing and PMS symptoms.

Your family doctor should be able to refer you to a therapist who practices cognitive therapy.

Meditation

Meditation is not really so much a therapy as a way of life. Once you have learnt how to meditate you will want to practise the technique every day – whether you're in good health or bad.

Meditation is not a 'religious' exercise, though many religions around the world use meditation to induce a feeling of peace and inner calm. Nor is it simply a case of sitting still for ten minutes. You need to learn to blot out the world so that you have a chance to listen to your 'inner self'.

If you haven't tried meditation before you may need a little practice before you get the hang of it, but you will. You can learn meditation by yourself at home but the best way is to join a class and get taught properly.

One of the simplest techniques involves the following steps:

- Sit with a straight back, either in a chair or cross-legged on the floor, with your hands resting in your lap and your feet firmly on the ground, feet slightly apart.
- Close your eyes and take several slow breaths – make sure your abdomen swells out when you breathe in and sinks back when you breathe out (it is hard to relax if you are breathing with your upper chest).

- Repeat a neutral word over and over again in your mind slowly – this word will be your 'mantra' (it can be any word but many people choose evocative ones such as 'one', 'peace' or 'flower').
- If you feel your mind wandering, and it is natural for it to do so, turn your mind back to your counting or your mantra.
- Do this for 15 minutes.
- At the end of that time stop and sit quietly for a minute or so before opening your eyes and getting up slowly.

Clinical research has shown that regular meditation can reduce stress levels and is of use in treating stress-related conditions. Patients treated for high blood pressure have even been able to reduce their medication after taking up meditation.

Autogenics

This is a cross between meditation, yoga and hypnotherapy and has to be taught in classes by a qualified teacher.

Often called 'passive concentration', autogenics teaches six basic mental exercises to help you switch off your stress response and switch on your relaxation and healing response. The exercises ask you to concentrate on your feelings of heaviness and warmth, your heartbeat and breathing, the warmth of your stomach and the coolness of your brow.

It is practised in three basic positions: sitting upright, the 'armchair position' and lying down. The idea is that as a result you can do the exercises anywhere – even going to work or sitting at a desk.

Creative visualization

If you've ever counted sheep to try and get to sleep then you have already used a form of creative visualization. It is a form of meditation in which you focus on an idea or an image.

You might think of a peaceful image such as a beautiful scene in the country to help you relax. Some people go further and picture images that 'take on' and beat their illness. A PMS sufferer might choose to imagine her PMS as a vivid red that she gradually changes to a soothing blue, for example.

The creative therapies

These include anything that you think you would enjoy, from painting, drawing, sculpture, and pottery to drama, gardening, dancing and so on. The aim is to express your emotions through a creative activity and to relax.

In painting therapy, for example, you might use colours to express your emotions. A technique using long, continuous brush strokes is associated with quiet, relaxed moods. Some people who are very introverted or shy may find that painting can give them the confidence to 'come out' of themselves.

The creative therapies are widely used in the treatment of patients with psychiatric conditions. They are not a cure but they can induce feelings of calmness and tranquillity which can only help.

Yoga

Yoga is a combination of mind and body therapy. It uses a series of physical poses – known as *asanas* – combined with breathing exercises – known as *pranayama* – to encourage physical and mental wellbeing.

Based on ancient Indian practice, the main aim is to improve the vital 'life force' or *prana* that is said to flow through you. You will not be expected to contort your body into impossible poses, but as your body becomes more supple you will find you will be able to perform more complicated poses naturally.

Because yoga is more of a philosophy than a therapy it is usually best taught by a qualified practitioner. There is little point in learning a few exercises from a book without understanding the thinking behind those exercises that will allow you to get the most out of them.

A yoga breathing exercise

The following breathing technique used in yoga will help you to relax. It should take about 15 minutes to do:

- Loosen clothing and take off your shoes. Lie on the floor, placing your arms by your side with the palms facing upwards. Spread your feet slightly apart and close your eyes.
- Lie quietly for a moment, breathing as you do normally. After a few minutes start to concentrate on how you are breathing. Are you a chest breather? Or do you breathe from the abdomen? How fast are you breathing?
- Slowly move your hands and place one on your chest and the other just below your rib cage. Now start to breathe in and out through your nose. As you breathe in your abdomen should rise upwards then sink down again when you breathe out. *Your chest should hardly move at all.*
- Give yourself a few minutes to learn to breathe with your abdomen. Focus on your breathing and let go of other thoughts that try and get in the way. If the thoughts intrude simply turn your attention back to your breathing and focus on its natural rhythm.
- Gradually your breathing will become calm and rhythmic as you become more relaxed. When you are ready, take a few deeper breaths, open your eyes and return to the world.

Abnormally deep or rapid breathing is known as *hyperventilation* and is a sign of anxiety. It is a common symptom of our hurried, stressful modern lives.

CHAPTER 9

Treating your body

Physical therapies for PMS

The aim of therapies which treat your body is to release your body's own natural powers of self-healing. The therapies described here are those most commonly used to treat PMS.

Acupuncture

One of the best known Chinese medicines is acupuncture. It has been used for thousands of years – archaeologists have even found primitive needles dating back to the Stone Age. Today, acupuncture is widely accepted in the West, particularly for pain relief.

The basic principles behind acupuncture are the same as those behind Chinese herbal medicine (see page 79). The central belief is that every living thing, like the universe as a whole, contains an energy or 'life force' called in Chinese *qi* (pronounced 'chee').

Illness is regarded as an upset of the *qi* and the aim is to restore the *qi* to its normal balance. So when you visit an acupuncturist he or she will first try to understand your *qi*.

The Chinese believe we inherit our *qi* and we maintain it throughout our life with what we eat and drink, and the air we breathe. They also believe *qi* changes according to your environment, the time of year, the weather, your diet, family circumstances and so on, so the acupuncturist will take all these factors into account during treatment.

The *qi* is believed to flow along a series of 'channels' – or *meridians* – in the body (*see* Figure 8). If there is a blockage in one of the 12 meridians the *qi* cannot flow properly and so the aim is to remove the blockage using acupuncture needles.

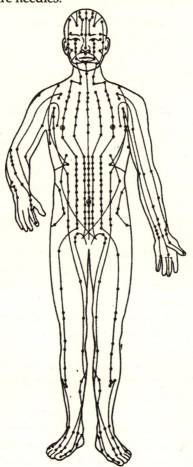

Fig. 8 The acupuncture 'energy' meridians and points

Chinese medicine uses a rather different system of diagnosis from that used in the West. First the practitioner will make a full record of your general health so that he or she can assess the state of your *qi*. Traditional methods of diagnosis include:

- the appearance and colour of your face
- the sound and quality of your voice
- the odour of your body
- the appearance of your skin
- your emotional state

Your tongue will also be closely examined for colour, shape and coating.

'Reading' your pulses has great significance in Chinese medicine and is more complicated than that used by Western medicine. The Chinese believe there are 12 pulses, six on each wrist, each of which is connected to 12 body regions. An experienced acupuncturist will be able to assess the state of your internal organs according to your pulses.

Once you have had a full examination the practitioner will group your symptoms according to one of eight set principles. These will class you as 'hot' or 'cold', 'dry' or 'damp' and so on.

A blockage of *qi* may cause an imbalance of the *yin* and the *yang* – the two opposite but complementary forces Chinese practitioners believe are in everyone. To be in good health *yin* and *yang* need to be in balance.

In addition to *yin* and *yang* Chinese medicine also has a system of elements. These improve or deteriorate according to the climate. The five elements are wood, fire, earth, metal and water. Each element relates to parts of the body: for example, wood is liver, gall bladder, tendons and eyes. An imbalance in the elements may lead to ill-health and can prevent healing.

PMS is regarded by acupuncturists as an imbalance in

the liver, particularly a 'stagnation' of the liver *qi*. A cause of abdominal bloating is stagnation of the *qi* in the lower abdomen.

Common PMS symptoms are closely associated with the liver. So irritability is associated with anger linked with the liver. Cravings for sugar are explained by excess liver energy which invades the spleen and causes deficiency and weakness.

To help clear stagnation in the liver *qi* needles will be inserted at various meridians. Treatment aims either to disperse the energy away from the needle site ('dispersion') or gather the energy towards the needle ('tonification').

Once inserted the needle is manipulated to tonify or disperse the energy. This usually takes less than 30 seconds. When energy is being dispersed the needle may be left in place for up to an hour and the practitioner will check the flow every so often by reading the pulses.

Some practitioners use 'moxibustion'. This is a technique that involves burning *moxa*, a dried herb (usually common mugwort), in one of various ways to apply a small degree of heat to the point needing treating.

Many people worry about having needles stuck into them but the needles used in acupuncture are so fine – barely wider than a human hair – that they are usually painless to insert and they are only inserted a few millimetres under the surface. Most people say they are hardly aware of them going in.

If you are worried about hygiene a good acupuncturist should use disposable needles that are only used on one person before being thrown away. Strict sterilization techniques should also be followed to prevent infection from one patient to another.

Herbal medicine

Plants have been used in healing since the very first humans walked the earth. Even today some of our most common medicines – aspirin, the oral contraceptive pill, and the heart drug *digitalis* for example – would not be here if it were not for traditional herbal remedies. Some of the latest developments in cancer treatment – such as *paclitaxel* (UK brand name Taxol), a drug derived from the yew tree used to treat ovarian cancer – are based on plants.

There are two main types of herbal medicine:

● Oriental, particularly Chinese
● Western

Chinese herbal medicine

Chinese herbalists use the same basic principles as those for acupuncture. Once again, the aim of the Chinese herbal practitioner treating PMS is to use herbs that stimulate and move the liver energy.

One of the most commonly used is *Paeonia lactiflora* (or *Bai Shao Yao* in Chinese). This is known to most people in the West as the common peony, a plant with large red, pink, white or yellow flowers we grow in our gardens. The root of this plant is believed to have a specific action on the liver, soothing the liver energy and improving its function. It also nourishes the blood and the *yin*.

Usually the plant is boiled up with water to make a 'tea'. It can also be mixed with other herbs such as licorice root, which is taken as a regular tonic.

Western herbal medicine

The principles of Western herbal medicine date back to the ancient Egyptians who used a range of herbs such as juniper, garlic, licorice and aloe vera to make medicines.

The ancient Greeks were heavily influenced by the

Egyptians and they devised a system of elements –
earth, air, fire and water – which were related to the four
bodily 'humours' or fluids, and four temperaments.

In a similar way to Chinese medicine, there were also
four categories of herbs – cold, hot, dry and damp –
which were used according to the type of patient.

Modern herbalism is built on these principles but a
modern herbalist is likely to understand much more
about the chemical and therapeutic effects of each herb
as science has helped to unravel exactly how herbs
work. Today herbs are grouped into categories according to their effect on the body:

- *Tonifying herbs* help to improve the body's ability to
  renew itself. They might stimulate certain organs or
  bodily processes such as the blood circulation.
- *Calming herbs* encourage relaxation which allows the
  body to recuperate from exertion or illness.
- *Eliminating herbs* help to cleanse the body, breaking
  down toxins that have built up.

Although many modern drugs are derived from plants,
herbalists believe that the plants in their natural state are
safer. To make modern drugs from plants a pharma-
ceutical company first analyses the active ingredient and
then extracts it, often developing a way of reproducing
its chemistry synthetically. The resulting drug is usually
therefore an artificial form of the active ingredient and
so pure and strong it is extremely toxic.

Herbalists say the plants they use contain hundreds,
even thousands, of other chemicals that act as a natural
'buffer' and 'balancer' to neutralize any harmful effects
of the active ingredients. Also herbal remedies often contain smaller amounts of the active dose which means
they are gentler therapies anyway, although they may
take longer to work.

There are two groups of herbs used in treating PMS:

- herbs that restore the hormone balance
- herbs that treat PMS symptoms

Herbs for hormone balance
Two of the most common are *Vitex agnus castus*, or chaste tree, and 'Pro-gest', a natural progesterone cream derived from the Mexican yam (*Dioscorea villosa*).

Vitex agnus castus is made from the berries of the chaste tree. It is thought to restore the correct balance of hormones by its action on the pituitary gland. A number of studies, mainly in Germany, have shown it is effective in treating PMS in some women. The herb is given as a liquid and the normal dose is 40 drops a day.

Pro-gest contains a substance called *diogenin* which is broken down by the body to produce progesterone. It was once used to produce the progesterone for the oral contraceptive pill before the days of chemically-synthesized hormones.

Pro-gest is supplied as a cream which is rubbed on to the skin twice a day during the second half of the cycle. The treatment has been criticized by conventional doctors who say it is difficult to measure how much of the hormone is being absorbed into the bloodstream using this method. But British expert Dr Peter Lewis, of the Centre for the Study of Complementary Medicine in Southampton, who has used both *agnus castus* and Pro-gest extensively for PMS, says that blood levels can be monitored, if necessary, by taking regular blood samples. In reality, he says, the patient's response to the therapy dictates how much of the drug is used. If symptoms are not relieved the dose is increased.

Pro-gest is an unlicensed medicine made by an American company – which means that in most countries it can only be prescribed by a qualified doctor. So you may need to visit a medically qualified herbalist for this therapy.

Some herbalists recommend a special hormone blend tea which contains *agnus castus* and Mexican yam as well as other ingredients such as ginseng, licorice, fennel, kelp, black cohosh, and false unicorn. The tea should be taken three times a day during the second half of the cycle for at least three months.

Herbs for PMS symptoms
PMS symptoms can be treated by the following herbs:

Depression and anxiety
Borage, lemon balm, chamomile, skullcap. Borage is one of the herbs most widely used to help psychological symptoms. A tea made of borage and lemon balm may be recommended for depression, while borage with chamomile and skullcap may be used for anxiety.

Breast pain and tenderness
Evening primrose oil (*see* Chapter 6).

Water retention
Diuretic herbs such as dandelion and cleavers are among the best but the range of diuretic herbs is very wide. The aim is to improve kidney function so that more water is excreted from the body to clean the blood and the lymphatic system. Usually you will be advised to take a tea containing a blend of herbs such as red clover, burdock and echinacea, as well as circulatory stimulants such as ginger or black pepper.

The leaves of the boldo plant are both a liver stimulant and a diuretic. Celery seeds and juniper berries may also be included for their diuretic properties. Remedies for PMS already widely available in good pharmacies or healthfood stores contain a mixture of boldo, celery and juniper.

Headaches

A wide variety of herbs can be used to treat headaches – though, generally, a herbalist will treat the background cause of the headache rather than simply doling out a remedy for the symptom.

One of the most common headache remedies is a tea containing one or more of the following herbs: meadowsweet, willowbark, poplar bark, lime flowers, peppermint, chamomile, rosemary, ginger, wood betony, basil, lemon balm, passion flower or sage.

Insomnia

Chamomile. Insomnia, inability to sleep, is often treated with chamomile tea. You can buy this yourself in most good stores. Other herbs which aid sleep are catnip, lemon balm, lime flowers, hops, lavender, wood betony, passion flower, skullcap and valerian.

You could also make a herbal pillow to help you sleep by filling a small muslin bag with a mixture of dried herbs from the above list and placing it in your pillow-case.

Caution Consult a qualified practitioner rather than trying to self-treat with herbs. It takes several years of training to build up the level of knowledge necessary to use herbs as medicines properly. Some plants used by herbalists, such as comfrey and valerian, can be highly toxic if not taken correctly.

Rosie's story

Rosie, a 34-year-old mother of three, went to see a herbalist on the advice of a friend: 'I'd always been very dismissive of women with PMS until I started suffering myself after the birth of my third baby. I had terrible postnatal depression which my doctor treated with antidepressants.

'About six months after that I kept getting really down just before my period. I felt as if life wasn't worth carrying on but then when my period started I'd cheer up and wonder how I could have been so stupid. I didn't want to go back on antidepressants so I tried this herbalist.

'He was really supportive. We went through all the things in my life that might be making the PMS worse, like my diet and looking after three young children. I began to feel better once I'd made my diet a bit healthier but it wasn't a complete answer – so he prescribed a herbal tea which I drank a couple of times a day in the two weeks before my period.

'It was great. By the second month I sailed through with hardly an off moment. I took the tea for six months and then because I felt I could cope I stopped and I've been fine ever since. I feel like the old me again'.

Nutrition therapy

In the past nutrition and herbalism went hand-in-hand. Plants we now regard as foods, such as fennel or lettuce, were eaten as much for their medicinal properties as their nutritional value.

Nutrition therapy, or nutritional medicine, is now a

widely-accepted treatment for PMS – even by conventional doctors. It is based on scientific evidence that:

- Many people have a low intake of essential nutrients, especially of vitamins and minerals.
- Needs for nutrients vary from one person to another so that what is an adequate intake for one person may not be for another.
- Illness may cause a biochemical abnormality which results in changes to the way vitamins and minerals are used by the body.
- Supplements of vitamins, minerals and essential fatty acids, combined with changes to diet, will correct biochemical abnormalities and restore a person to good health.
- Correcting nutritional deficiencies will improve symptoms and prevent disease.

An organization in Britain that specializes in this approach is the Women's Nutritional Advisory Service (WNAS) in Hove, southern England. WNAS claims to have helped more than 90 per cent of the women who have contacted it with PMS problems. Run by a nutritionist and a medical doctor qualified in nutritional medicine, it offers a worldwide postal service as well as personal consultations (*see* Appendix A).

The main therapy is dietary change, based on healthy eating principles as outlined in Chapter 4. Many women are also prescribed a dietary supplement containing B vitamins (including B6), magnesium and other trace elements that may be missing from the diet.

Homoeopathy

Homoeopathy is one of the natural medicines that gets conventional doctors particularly upset. The remedies it uses are so dilute that many doctors feel there is no known scientific way that they can possibly work. But many patients swear by its effectiveness and there is a growing band of medically-qualified homoeopaths.

Homoeopathy is an approach to the treatment of disease completely different from conventional medicine, based on the findings of a German doctor, Samuel Hahnemann, in the early 1800s.

Hahnemann discovered that substances that produce certain symptoms in healthy people could be used to treat sick people who already had those symptoms. For example, the malaria treatment Peruvian bark produced symptoms of malaria when he ate it. This led to his principle of 'let like be cured by like'.

One of the problems in the early days was that the remedies often made sick people even sicker so Hahnemann tried diluting them. To his surprise he found they were more effective when they were diluted.

Today over 3,000 remedies are used by homoeopaths. They come from plant, animal or mineral sources which are ground down and then diluted in a solution of alcohol and water before being vigorously shaken. The shaking, or 'succussion' is said by homoeopaths to be just as important as the diluting. The result is taken as a liquid or converted into tablets dissolved in the mouth.

Like the other natural remedies, homoeopathy is based on the idea that a person's natural healing abilities need to be released. A first consultation with a homoeopath is likely to last at least an hour and will concentrate on you as the individual. You will be classified according to your constitution and a remedy will be made up to suit you.

Some typical PMS remedies include pulsatilla, calcarea, sepia, lycopodium, sulphur, natrum mur, nux vom, and phosphorus.

If you experienced premenstrual headaches, irritability, confusion and depression you might be prescribed sepia, for example. Someone with irritability combined with anxiety, anger, hot flushes and cravings for sugar may be more suited to sulphur.

Often symptoms get worse before they get better – this is known as the 'aggravation reaction' – and it shows that the treatment is working.

You might be advised by the homoeopath to avoid certain foods and drinks while on your course of therapy. Strong foods such as peppermint, coffee and chilli, for example, may interfere with the remedy and are usually to be avoided.

Flower remedies

One of the best-known self-treatments for PMS is flower remedies. The most famous are the 'Bach Remedies' – named after their founder Dr Edward Bach, a British homoeopath who devised a range of 39 remedies early this century from the wild flowers and plants growing around his Oxfordshire home – but there are now versions made and sold in both America and Australia.

A sort of cross between homoeopathy and herbalism, flower remedies claim to work by treating psychological conditions. For example, the Bach remedy mustard (*Sinapsis arvensis*) is used to treat depression and sadness while holly (*Ilex aquifolium*) is for negative feelings such as suspicion, jealousy and hatred.

The most widely-used Bach remedy is 'Rescue Remedy' – a five-flower mixture of rock rose (terror and fear), impatiens (agitation, irritability and inability to relax), clematis (absent-mindedness), Star of Bethlehem (stress after a traumatic experience), and cherry plum (losing emotional and physical control). It is said to be useful for relief during stressful situations and major crises or moments of anxiety.

There have been no clinical studies to support the claims made for flower remedies but thousands of women around the world swear by them for PMS nevertheless.

Naturopathy

Naturopathy is based on the principle that the human body has an inbuilt healing ability. A naturopath believes that because the body has the capacity to heal a cut or mend a broken bone it also has the capacity – with a little help – to heal other disorders.

'Pure' naturopathy was originally known as 'Nature Cure' or 'Natural Hygiene' and a few practitioners who practise this form still call it this. The basic approach is to eat pure food, breathe pure air and drink pure water. Diet should be wholefood and high fibre, and preferably organically grown and free of all additives.

Modern naturopaths supplement diet with vitamins and minerals but 'old school' naturopaths frown upon the use of supplements preferring to use wholesome foods instead. Both old and new naturopaths believe in hydrotherapy (water therapy) procedures such as hot and cold baths, spa baths, and mud packs to help rid the body of toxins. Some naturopaths also recommend fasting or a diet of one food such as grapes to clear the body of toxins. This treatment is not generally recommended for women with PMS who may already have problems with low blood sugar.

In most countries (Britain is an exception) modern naturopaths are trained in a wide range of natural therapies including acupuncture, homoeopathy, herbalism and osteopathy, and are the 'general practitioners' of natural medicine, comparable to conventional doctors.

Aromatherapy and massage

If you fall over and bump yourself the first instinct is to rub it better – and that is the basic idea behind massage. There are several 'schools' of massage but the main principles are the same.

In massage the soft tissues of the body – the muscles and ligaments – are rubbed and manipulated to ease tensions, improve circulation and stimulate the lymphatic system, which helps get rid of the body's waste material.

Aromatherapy uses massage as the basis of therapy with the addition of 'essential oils' – oils distilled from plants – to help healing and prevent disease. As well as smelling very nice, essential oils are thought to have medicinal properties and are used in a variety of ways:

- as massage oils
- added to the bath
- heated in a special burner to release fragrance into a room
- inhaled as a few drops on a handkerchief
- added (one or two drops only) to a drink

Our sense of smell is highly developed and everyone has at least one smell that can bring a memory flooding back – such as the image of school conjured up by the odour of boiled cabbage! Aromatherapists, however, believe that essential oils have healing powers, particularly when they're used as part of a whole body treatment that includes diet and stress reduction.

There is evidence for the healing power of oils as far back as 1928 when one of the pioneers of aromatherapy, a French chemist called René Gattefosse, published an account of how he had burnt his hand in a laboratory explosion at the perfumery where he worked. He had plunged his hand into a bowl of lavender oil and had been amazed at how quickly it had healed – with no sign of scarring.

Even conventional medicine is recognizing the benefits of aromatherapy. In the UK several state National Health Service hospitals employ aromatherapists, particularly in midwifery, children's wards and in the care of the elderly and cancer patients.

Home remedies for PMS include oils of ylang ylang, lavender or clary sage added to a nightly bath taken in the second half of the menstrual cycle. A few drops of clary sage on a handkerchief may be handy to prevent weepiness. Juniper oil added to the bath may ease water retention.

The nice thing about aromatherapy is that it's a very flexible therapy. You can pay to see a specialist aroma-therapist – preferably one trained in the proper thera-peutic use of oils rather than just a beauty therapist – or you can do it yourself at home with the help of a good aromatherapy book.

Reflexology

Reflexology is another therapy said to have ancient, possibly Chinese, origins. It involves manipulating specific 'pressure points' on the soles and sides of the feet that therapists claim represent different parts of the body.

The technique was rediscovered in the West in the 1920s when an American surgeon discovered that he could make his ear go numb by applying pressure to a certain part of his foot. The effect was so strong that he could perform minor ear operations while the patient's foot was being manipulated.

According to reflexologists, the sole of the foot is a map of the whole body. The right foot represents the right side of the body and the left foot the left side. So the big toes represent the head and brain and the heart is represented by the area just above the middle of the left foot. The reflex points associated with PMS symptoms are shown in Figure 9.

The aim of reflexology is to put pressure on the area of the foot that corresponds to the part of the body that needs treatment. The pressure is thought to stimulate the

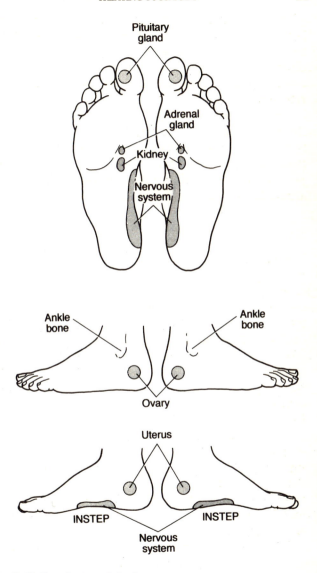

Fig. 9 Reflexology points for PMS

body's natural healing powers, possibly by removing blocks to the free flow of *qi* as in acupuncture. Another explanation is that it helps improve blood circulation and reduces tension.

There are no harmful side-effects of reflexology. Sometimes symptoms may get worse for a few days, or you may develop a skin rash or need to pass water more often. Natural therapists call this a 'healing crisis' and believe it is a sign that the body is healing itself by getting rid of toxins.

The hands, too, are believed to have reflex areas, although it is easier to treat the feet as they are bigger and more sensitive. Other reflex points, known as 'cross reflexes', are said to occur in other parts of the body linking the hip and shoulder, elbow and knee and the wrist and ankle.

A modern 'hi-tech' form of reflexology known as Vacuflex is said to be particularly effective in PMS. Developed in Denmark, it claims to achieve better results quicker by the use of special felt boots and a system of suction pads. Air is drawn out of the boots by a pump and the feet given an 'all-over' squeeze by the vacuum created. The suction pads are then used in much the same way as in the Chinese technique of 'cupping' to stimulate various reflex points on the feet, legs, arms and hands.

US research shows reflexology can help PMS

A study in America of 35 women with PMS showed that reflexology can significantly reduce symptoms of the condition.

Dr Terry Oleson and William Flocco from the Division of Behavioral Medicine and the American Academy of Reflexology, both in California, studied a group of women who were treated with reflexology on the points thought to be linked with PMS. Another group of women had dummy or 'placebo' reflexology: they still had the massage but it was on points that were not associated with PMS.

Both groups had weekly sessions for two months and were then followed up for a further two months. At the end of the treatment period the reflexology group showed a 46 per cent reduction in total PMS symptoms compared with 19 per cent for the placebo group.

Even two months after the treatment had finished there was a significant reduction in PMS scores in the treatment group compared with the placebo group. All of the women found the treatment relaxing and pleasant, even if they were only having the dummy massage.

The researchers admit that reductions in PMS symptoms were not as great as those seen in studies of relaxation (*see* Chapter 5) or for medical treatments. But the technique may be useful as part of a whole programme of PMS therapy or for women with mild to moderate PMS who do not want medical treatment.

CHAPTER 10

How to find and choose a natural therapist

Tips and guidelines for finding reliable help

It is much easier now to find the right therapist than it was even a few years ago – but it is still not easy enough. The sheer variety of therapies is bewildering in itself and in many countries natural therapists are still not fully organized. There is no shortage of directories and advertisements but it is difficult to know who to rely on for what from lists alone. So how do you find a therapist you can trust?

Starting the search: local sources

As we have seen, many of the natural therapies highlighted in this book have their roots in antiquity. Some have existed for as long as human beings have lived on earth, and finding a good practitioner has been a matter of tuning in to the community 'bush telegraph'. Word of mouth is still the best way to find the right practitioner.

Speak to anyone whose opinion you respect, especially if he or she is also a fellow sufferer. (You will also want to know who should be avoided, and which therapies might not help you at all.) If this does not work there are several other ways you can try:

Doctors' clinics and medical centres

If you need help urgently you must see your family doctor. It has already been explained in this book that your condition can decline quickly without the proper treatment. If you ask about natural therapies at your first appointment, be prepared to hear anything from a dire warning to a recommendation that you might try a natural therapist once your condition is stable.

Natural health centres

Your nearest natural health centre should be happy to advise you. Your first impressions will often be a good guide to the quality of service they provide. Are the staff well informed and friendly? Is the place clean and comfortable? Does the atmosphere make you feel comfortable from the moment you walk in? It should. It matters. You are bringing them your trust and your custom and both should be treated with the utmost respect.

A good centre should have plenty of information explaining the therapies and introducing the practitioners. In a well-run practice the receptionist or owner will know all about the different therapies on offer. It's a bad sign if they don't.

You may still be unsure after your first impressions whether to book in or not. If so, ask to meet the person who might be treating you, just to test the waters. This should be possible, even in a busy practice.

Don't start off by telling your full life history, but some practices do offer you this opportunity during a free consultation – usually 15 minutes – just to see whether you have come to the right place or not.

Local practitioners

Practitioners tend to know who's who in the area, even in therapies other than their own. So if you know, say, a reflexologist, but want a homoeopath, ask for a recommendation. The same applies if you know a practitioner socially and so don't want to consult him or her professionally. Practitioners are usually happy to recommend someone else in the same field.

Healthfood stores and alternative bookshops
The staff in these kinds of shops often have a good local knowledge as well as an interest in the subject of natural therapies. The shop may well have a noticeboard with local practitioners' business cards on it. Remember, though, the most experienced and well-established practitioners don't need this kind of advertising, so you might miss them altogether if you don't actually check up by asking.

Other sources of local knowledge
Don't forget that your local pharmacist often has contacts with both conventional and natural therapists.

The local library or information centre may be another good source of contact, especially for finding self-help or support groups.

Computers (using a modem) can provide this type of information via the Internet system and other sources worth trying are health farms, beauty therapists and citizens' advice bureaux.

Wider sources of information

If you have no luck on a local level, don't give up – there are several more leads you can follow up at a national level.

'Umbrella' organizations
The natural therapies are increasingly coming together under 'umbrella' organizations that represent a therapy or range of therapies nationally under one banner or heading. These national umbrella organizations have lists of registered and approved practitioners, and in the

case of the more established therapies (such as chiropractic) have their own regulatory bodies already in place.

It is better to phone than to write or fax because this should give you a good idea of how well organized the group is. You may find that the group you are contacting has several different associations under its banner. A small charge may be made for each association's register but if you can afford it get the lot and then make up your own mind.

Newspapers, magazines and local directories
Many therapists advertise. If you find local practitioners this way it's a good idea to talk to them and check them out first.

Checking professional organizations

Some organizations are genuine groups that really keep a check on their members, while others seem to spring up like weeds, apparently interested only in collecting membership fees and giving themselves credibility. This section helps you do your own weeding.

Why do professional organizations exist?
The purposes of governing bodies for natural therapies are:

● to keep up-to-date lists of their members so you can check whether someone is really on their list or not
● to protect you by making sure that their members are fully trained, licensed and insured against accident, negligence and malpractice
● to give you someone to complain to if you are unhappy with any aspect of treatment you have received, and you can't sort the matter out with your therapist
● to protect their members by giving good ethical and legal advice

- to represent their members when laws which might affect them are being made
- to work towards improvements in education for their members both before and after qualifying
- to work towards greater awareness of the benefit of each therapy in conventional medical circles
- to improve public awareness of the benefit of each therapy

Questions to ask professional organizations

A good organization will publish clear and simple information on its status and purposes along with its membership list. As they don't all do this you may find it useful to contact them again on receiving your list to ask the following:

- When was the association founded? (You may be reassured to hear it has been around for 50 years. If the association is new, however, don't reject it out of hand. Ask why it was formed – it may be innovative.)
- How many members does it have? (Size reflects public demand, as few therapists could survive in a therapy if there was no call for it. The bigger organizations generally have a better track record and greater public acceptance, but a small association may just reflect the fact that the therapy is very specialized or still in its infancy – not necessarily a bad thing.)
- When was the therapy that it represents started?
- Is it a charity or educational trust – with a proper constitution, management committee, and published accounts – or is it a private limited company? (Charities have to be non-profitmaking, work in the public interest, and be open to inspection at any time. Private companies don't.)
- Is it part of a larger network of organizations? (If so, this implies it is interested in progress by consensus with other groups, and not just in furthering its own

aims. By and large, groups that go their own way are more suspect than those that join in.)

- Does the organization have a code of ethics (upholding standards of professional behaviour) and disciplinary procedures? If so, what are they?
- How do its members gain admission to its register? Is it linked to only one school? (Beware of associations whose heads are also head of the school they represent: unbiased help may be in short supply with this type of 'one man band'.)
- Do members have to have proof of professional indemnity insurance? This should cover:
  - accidental damage to yourself or your property while you are on the practitioner's work premises
  - negligence (either the failure of the practitioner to exercise the 'duty of care' owed to you, or his or her falling below the standards of clinical competence demanded by his or her qualifications, bringing about an overall worsening of your problem)
  - malpractice (a 'falling from grace' over professional conduct, involving, for example, dishonesty, sexual misconduct or breach of confidence – your personal details should *never* be discussed with a third person without your permission)

Checking training and qualifications

If you have reassured yourself so far but are still puzzled by what the training actually involves, ask a few more questions:

- How long is the training?
- Is it full- or part-time?
- If it is part-time but shorter than a full-time course leading to the same qualifications, does the time spent at lectures and in clinic add up to the same as a full-time course overall? (In other words, is it a short cut?)

- Does it include seeing patients under supervision at a college clinic and in real practices?
- What do the initials after the therapist's name mean? Do they denote simply membership of an organization or do they indicate in-depth study?
- Are the qualifications recognized? If so, by whom? (This is becoming more relevant as the therapy organizations group together and start to form state-recognized registers in many countries. But the really important thing to know is if the qualifications are recognized by an independent outside assessment authority.)

Making the choice

Making the final choice is a matter of using a combination of common sense and intuition, and finding the resolution to give someone a try. Don't forget that the most important part of the whole process is your resolve to feel better, to have more control over your state of health, and hopefully to see an improvement in your condition. The next most important part is that you feel comfortable with your chosen therapist.

What is it like seeing a natural therapist?

Since most natural therapists, even in those countries with state health systems, still work privately, there is no established common pattern.

Although they may all share more or less a belief in the principles outlined in chapter 7, you are liable to come across individuals from all walks of life. You will find as much variety in dress, thinking and behaviour as there are fashions, ranging from the formal and sophisticated to the absolutely informal.

Equally, you will find their premises very different.

Some will present a 'brass plaque' image, working in a clinic with a receptionist and brisk efficiency, while others will see you in their living room surrounded by plants and domestic clutter.

Remember, though, that while image may be some indication of status, it is little guarantee of ability. You are as likely to find a therapist of quality working from home as in a formal clinic.

Some characteristics, though, and probably the most important ones, are common to all natural therapists:

- They will give you far more time than you are used to with a family doctor. An initial consultation will rarely last less than an hour, and is often longer. They will ask you all about yourself so they can form a proper understanding of what makes you tick and what may be the fundamental cause(s) of your problem.
- You will have to pay for any remedies they prescribe, and they may well sell you these from their own stocks. They will also charge you for their time – though many therapists offer reduced fees for deserving cases or for people who genuinely cannot afford the full fee.

Sensible precautions

- Be sceptical of anyone who 'guarantees' you a cure. No one (not even doctors) can do that.
- Query any attempt to book you in for a course of treatment. Your response to any natural therapy is highly individual. Of course, if the practice is a busy one, booking ahead for one or two sessions might be sensible. You should be able to cancel without penalty any sessions which prove unnecessary (but remember to give at least 24 hours' notice: some practitioners will charge you if you don't give enough notice).

- No ethical therapist will ask for fees in advance of treatment unless for special tests or medicines – and even this is unusual. If you are asked for 'down payments' of any sort, ask exactly what they are for. If you don't like the reasons, don't pay.
- Be wary if you are not asked about your existing medication, and try to give precise answers when you are asked. Be especially wary if the therapist tells you to stop or change any medically prescribed drug without talking to your doctor first. (A responsible doctor should also be happy to discuss you and your medication with a therapist.)
- Note the quality of the therapist's touch if you choose any of the relaxation or manipulation techniques such as massage, aromatherapy or osteopathy. It should never be lingering or suggestive. If, for any reason, the therapist wants to touch you on the breasts or genitals, your permission should be sought first.
- If the practitioner is of the opposite sex you are entitled to have someone of your choice in the room at the same time. Be immediately suspicious if this is not allowed. Ethical therapists will not refuse this sort of request, and if they do, it is probably best to have nothing more to do with them.

What to do if things go wrong

A practitioner is in a position of trust, and is charged with a duty of care to you at all times. It does not mean you are 'entitled' to a 'cure' just because you've paid for treatment, but if you feel you are being treated unfairly, incompetently or unethically, you have several options:

- Tackle the matter at the source of the problem, with your practitioner, either verbally or in writing.
- If he or she works in a place such as a clinic, health

farm or sports centre, tell the management. They also have a duty to protect the public and should treat complaints seriously and discreetly.

- Contact the practitioner's professional organization. It should have an independent panel that investigates complaints fully and disciplines its members.
- If the offence committed is a criminal one report it to the police (but be prepared for the problem of proving one person's word against another's).
- If you feel compensation is due see a lawyer for advice.

Short of a public court case, the worst thing for a truly incompetent or unethical practitioner is bad publicity. Tell everyone about your experiences. People only need to hear the same sort of comments from a few different sources and the practitioner will probably sink without trace. Before you do so, though, try the other measures first and give yourself time to consider things calmly. Vengeance is not very healing.

A word of warning Don't make malicious allegations without good reason. Such actions are themselves a criminal offence in most countries and you could end up in more trouble than the practitioner.

Summary

The reality is that there are few real crooks or charlatans in natural therapy. Despite the myth, there is little real money in it unless the therapist is very busy – and the chances are high that a busy therapist is a good one. Remember that no one can know everything and no specialist qualified in any field has to get 100 per cent in the exams to be able to practise. Perfection is an ideal, not a reality, and to err is human.

It is very much for this reason that taking control of your own health is perhaps the single most important lesson underlying this book. Taking control means taking responsibility for the choices you make, and this is one of the most significant factors in successful treatment.

No one but you can decide on a practitioner and no-one but you can determine if that practitioner is any good or not. You will know this very easily, and probably very quickly, by the way you feel about the person and the therapy, and by whether or not you get any better.

If you are not happy, the decision is yours whether to stay or move on – and continue moving until you find the right therapist for you. Don't despair if you don't find the right person first time. There is almost bound to be the right person for you somewhere and your determination to get well is the best resource you have for finding that person.

Above all, bear in mind that many people who have taken this route before you have not only been helped beyond their most optimistic dreams, but have also found a close and trusted helper who will assist in times of trouble – and who may even become a friend for life.

APPENDIX A

Useful organizations

The following list of organizations is for information only and does not imply any endorsement, nor do the organizations listed necessarily agree with the views expressed in this book.

INTERNATIONAL

International Federation of Practitioners of Natural Therapeutics
10 Copse Close
Sheet
Petersfield
Hampshire GU31 4DL, UK.
Tel 01730 266790
Fax 01730 260058

AUSTRALASIA

Australian Natural Therapists Association
PO Box 308
Melrose Park
South Australia 5039.
Tel 8297 9533
Fax 8297 0003

Australian Traditional Medicine Society
PO Box 442
Suite 3, First Floor,
120 Blaxland Road
Ryde
New South Wales 2112.
Tel 2808 2825
Fax 2809 7570

New Zealand Natural Health Practitioners Accreditation Board
PO Box 37–491
Auckland.
Tel 9625 9966

Premenstrual Support Group of Victoria
9 Quixley Grove
Wantirna
Victoria 3131, Australia.
Tel 9801 2001

Womanline
Women's Health Centre
63 Ponsonby Road
Auckland
New Zealand.
Tel 9376 5173

NORTH AMERICA

American Holistic Medical Association
6728 Old McLean Village Drive
McLean, VA 22101, USA
Tel 703 556 9222

Canadian Holistic Medical Association
700 Bay Street
PO Box 101, Suite 604
Toronto
Ontario M5G 1Z6, Canada.
Tel 416 599 0447

Pre-menstrual Syndrome Centre
1077 North Service Road
Applewood Plaza
Mississauga
Ontario K0A 3G0, Canada.
Tel 416 273 7770

SOUTH AFRICA

South Africa Homoeopaths, Chiropractors and Allied Professions Board
PO Box 17055
0027 Groenkloof.
Tel 2712 466 455

UK and EIRE

Some of the UK-based groups offer a postal service to PMS sufferers in other countries.
Association for Post-natal Illness
7 Gowan Avenue
London SW6 6RH, UK.
Tel 0171-731 4867

British Association for Counselling
1 Regent Place
Rugby
Warwickshire CV21 2PJ, UK.
Tel 01788 578328

British Holistic Medical Association
Royal Shrewsbury Hospital
South
Shrewsbury
Shropshire SY3 8XF, UK.
Tel 01743 261155
Fax 01743 353637

British Society of Medical and Dental Hypnosis
42 Links Road
Ashtead
Surrey KT21 1HJ, UK.
Tel 01372 273522

Council for Complementary and Alternative Medicine
179 Gloucester Place
London NW1 6DW, UK.
Tel 0171-724 9103

Institute for Complementary Medicine
PO Box 194
London SE16 1QZ, UK.
Tel 0171-237 5165

National Association for PMS (NAPS)
PO Box 72
Sevenoaks
Kent TN13 1XQ, UK.
Tel 01732 459378

PMS Help
PO Box 160
St Albans
Herts AL1 4UQ, UK.
Postal enquiries only (send sae)

The Premenstrual Society
(PREMSOC)
PO Box 429
Addlestone
Surrey KT15 1DZ, UK.
Postal enquiries only (send sae)

Women's Health Concern
83 Earl's Court Road
London W8 6EF, UK.
Tel 0171-938 3932

Women's Health Information
Centre
52-54 Featherstone Street
London EC1Y 8RT, UK.
Tel 0171-251 6580

Women's Nutritional Advisory
Service
PO Box 268
Hove
East Sussex BN3 1RW, UK.
Tel 01273 487366

Useful further reading

Acupuncture, Peter Mole (Element, UK, 1992)

Aromatherapy, Christine Wildwood (Element, UK, 1991)

Beat PMT through Diet, Maryon Stewart (Ebury Press, UK, 1988)

The Complete Yoga Course, Howard Kent (Headline Press, UK, 1993)

Coping with Periods, Diana Saunders (Chambers, UK, 1985)

Encyclopaedia of Natural Medicine, Brian Inglis and Ruth West (Michael Joseph, UK, 1983)

The Handbook of Complementary Medicine, Stephen Fulder (Oxford Medical Publications, UK, 1988)

Nutritional Medicine, Stephen Davies and Alan Stewart (Pan Books, UK, 1987)

Seeing Red: The Politics of Premenstrual Tension, S Laws, V Hey and A Eagan (Hutchinson, UK, 1986)

Self Help with PMS, Michelle Harrison (MacDonald, UK, 1990)

The Women's Guide to Homoeopathy, Andrew Lockie and Nicola Geddes (Hamish Hamilton, UK, 1992)

Index

BHMA TAPES FOR HEALTH

*Practical self-help packages designed by
experts to make taking care of yourself easier*

Imagery For Relaxation by Duncan Johnson
Exercises in visualization to help relaxation and influence the functions
of the body and mind. To provide yourself with the opportunity to
learn more about your attitudes and neglected needs. To harness the
forces of the creative mind and change negative attitudes to life.

Getting To Sleep by Ashley Conway
A practical help with insomnia. Promotes relaxation and positive
thinking to put you in touch with your body's 'normal' sleep pattern.

Introduction To Meditation by Dr Sarah Eagger
This tape is a progressive learning programme of meditation exercises.
Teaching you how to begin using meditation for increasing your peace
of mind and well-being.

Coping With Persistent Pain by Dr James Hawkins
Teaches relaxation skills in a greater depth, and how to apply those
skills as a coping method during daily activities. To help promote
some form of normality into a life of constant pain.

Coping With Stress by Dr David Peters
A programme to teach you how to build the relaxation response into
your life. Understanding stress and dealing with it through relaxation
techniques.

The Breath Of Life by Dr Patrick Pietroni
A muscular relaxation technique which explores the connection
between stress and our breathing rhythm. With exercises on how to
control breathing to alleviate symptoms of stress.

Please write to the British Holistic Medical Association at Rowland
Thomas House, Royal Shrewbury Hospital South, Shrewsbury,
Shropshire, SY3 8XF for full details of tapes and mail order service.